3D/4D Printing of Bioadhesive Pharmaceutical Systems

This book features a brief history of additive manufacturing and 3D/4D printing techniques, as well as the advantages, applications, and overall challenges facing the technology. It then focuses on the applications of bioadhesive systems for drug delivery.

3D/4D Printing of Bioadhesive Pharmaceutical Systems: Additive Manufacturing and Perspectives explores recent discoveries of 3D printing in the development of pharmaceutical systems and drug delivery. Specifically, it discusses the main polymers/materials used in the development of bio-adhesive pharmaceutical systems and explains the importance of bioadhesiveness of drug release through 3D printing. The authors also introduce the main strategies necessary to achieve a proper drug delivery system through 3D printing, and examine the adhesiveness of these systems on the skin as the mucosa decreases with the elimination of the drug by the body. Finally, the book brings all the necessary specifications to obtain a bioadhesive system with suitable bio-ink to obtain the best 3D/4D printing.

This book is written with the objective of helping students start their studies in pharmaceutical engineering, bioengineering, and additive manufacturing. Moreover, engineering professionals can use the book to improve the performance of 3D/4D printers for this type of system.

3D/4D Printing
of Bioadhesive
Pharmaceutical Systems

Additive Manufacturing and Perspectives

Marcos Luciano Bruschi, Denise Tiemi Uchida,
and Mariana Carla de Oliveira

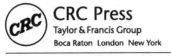

CRC Press
Taylor & Francis Group
Boca Raton London New York

CRC Press is an imprint of the
Taylor & Francis Group, an **informa** business

Designed cover image: © Shutterstock

First edition published 2025
by CRC Press
2385 NW Executive Center Drive, Suite 320, Boca Raton FL 33431

and by CRC Press
4 Park Square, Milton Park, Abingdon, Oxon, OX14 4RN

CRC Press is an imprint of Taylor & Francis Group, LLC

© 2025 Marcos Luciano Bruschi, Denise Tiemi Uchida, and Mariana Carla de Oliveira

ISBN: 978-1-032-57926-9 (hbk)
ISBN: 978-1-032-58064-7 (pbk)
ISBN: 978-1-003-44236-3 (ebk)

DOI: 10.1201/9781003442363

Typeset in Times
by Deanta Global Publishing Services, Chennai, India

Contents

About the Authors

Marcos Luciano Bruschi is an Associate Professor in the Department of Pharmacy at the State University of Maringa (UEM), Parana, Brazil. Dr. Bruschi joined the university in 1998 as Assistant Professor of Pharmaceutics and became Associate Professor in 2014. He was awarded the degree of Doctor in Pharmaceutical Sciences from School of Pharmacy, University of Sao Paulo (USP), Brazil, with a period as a research fellow at Queen's University of Belfast (QUB), Northern Ireland, UK. In 2014, he returned to QUB complete a period of post-doctoral studies in School of Pharmacy. His current research focuses on the development of drug delivery systems using different strategies to modify and control drug delivery, including nanotechnology and the development of advanced thermoresponsive bioadhesive platforms, micro/nanostructured particles, 3D printing, natural products, and photodynamic therapy. He is the coordinator of the Laboratory of Research and Development of Drug Delivery Systems (LABSLiF) at the State University of Maringa.

Denise Tiemi Uchida is a PhD student in Pharmaceutical Sciences working on the development of bioadhesive drug delivery systems by 3D printing in the Laboratory of Research and Development of Drug Delivery Systems (LABSLiF) at the State University of Maringa, Brazil.

Mariana Carla de Oliveira is a PhD student in Pharmaceutical Sciences working on the development of controlled drug delivery systems in the Laboratory of Research and Development of Drug Delivery Systems (LABSLiF) at the State University of Maringa, Brazil.

1 Introduction to Additive Manufacturing

From History to Application

1.1 TIMELINE

Additive manufacturing (AM) or three-dimensional (3D) printing is a process that is capable of printing an object in 3D, regardless of size or format. In recent years, AM has grown rapidly and has been gaining space in various commercial and biomedical areas.

AM is nothing more than an evolution of 2D printing. The main difference being that in AM the ink or filament is deposited layer by layer until it forms a desired structure with three dimensions: length, width, and height.

Even as 3D printing is gaining notoriety, 4D printing is also currently emerging. In this additional dimension, the structure begins to change its geometric shape (morphology) in the face of a specific external stimulus, such as thermal, chemical, physical, among others stimuli, in a reversible or non-reversible manner, which will be covered in more detail in Chapter 6.

The first 3D printer prototypes appeared in the 1980s, but it was in the mid-1990s that manufacturers began to produce this technology for commercial use. The great inventor of this technology was Charles Hull, also known as the father of 3D Printing (Gokhare, Raut, and Shinde 2017; Wohlers and Gornet 2016). He developed this technology while working at his startup, 3D System Corporation, and the first 3D printer developed was the stereolithography (SLA) system.

The stereolithography 3D printer was the starting point for new types of 3D printers to be created over time (Figure 1.1). SLA, invented by Charles Hull, uses a photocurable resin to print the desired product. With this new invention, a variety of materials began to be printed in 3D such as biomaterials, food, plastics, metals, ceramics, among others (Hager, Golonka, and Putanowicz 2016; Han et al. 2023; Koide et al. 1993; X. Li et al. 2020; Wang et al. 2022; Zheng et al. 2019).

In the course of history, it can be said that 3D printing has gone through about five stages up to the present day (Prashar, Vasudev, and Bhuddhi 2022). The first phase that occurred in the 1970s and 1980s was marked by isolated occasions that may be indicative of being precursors of AM technology. The second phase was remarkable as it was the the beginning of AM, it occurred in the mid-1980s to the 1990s and was when the creation and launch of AM took place. The third phase, a little larger than the others, occurred around 1990 to 2005. In this phase, we can notice the

DOI: 10.1201/9781003442363-1

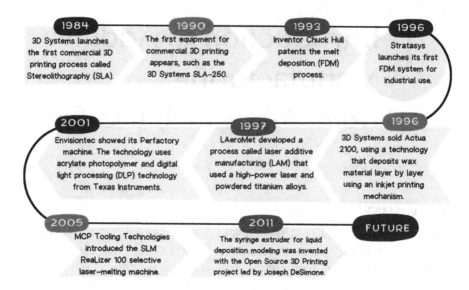

FIGURE 1.1   History of additive manufacturing (AM). A timeline reporting the main 3D printers developed.

maturation of this technology as well as its advancement, the progress of software, image resolution, and the emergence of new types of printing in 3D.

The third phase is also marked by the emergence of private companies manufacturing and using AM. The fourth phase, from 2005 to 2012, coincides with the expiration of authentic AM patents and the adoption of social media to propagate this technology. The fourth phase was marked by the acceptance and use of this technology by the general population.

The fifth phase (2012 onwards) marks the breakthrough and popularity of 3D printing. During this period, new 3D printing technologies emerged, and various printable materials were developed. It was in the fifth phase that AM became popular in the scientific community and began to receive funding, making it possible to acquire these technologies for research.

1.2   APPLICATIONS

In recent decades, additive manufacturing, also known as 3D and/or 4D printing, has been applied in a wide range of industries such as the food industry, the pharmaceutical and biomedical industry, and the civil construction industry, where it is used to produce various accessories such as costume jewelry and souvenirs.

Production flexibility and obtaining a functional structure with precise mechanical properties were characteristics that led to the application of AM in several areas. AM can be used in various fields as it is capable of printing various parts with complex structures (Table 1.1).

TABLE 1.1

Types of Printers and Their Application for Various Industrial Fields

Industrial Fields	3D Printer	Applications	Reference(s)
Biomedical	Fused deposition modeling 3D printer	Splint	(J. Li and Tanaka 2018)
	Digital light processing	Bone tissue scaffolds	(Liu et al. 2019; Rajput et al. 2022)
	Digital light processing	Artificial skin	(Choi et al. 2023)
	Inkjet	Tissue engineering	(Cui et al. 2012)
	Extrusion	Tissue engineering	(Hospodiuk et al. 2018)
Food	Extrusion	Food material	(Mantihal, Kobun, and Lee 2020; Rando and Ramaioli 2021; Yang et al. 2018)
Pharmaceutical	Stereolithographic	Oral drug delivery	(Wang et al. 2016)
	Inkjet-based	Wound Healing	(Albanna et al. 2019)
	Digital light processing	Microneedles	(Shin and Hyun 2021)
	Stereolithographic	Microneedles	(Farias et al. 2018)
	Two-photon polymerisation	Microneedles	(Cordeiro et al. 2020)

In the food sector, AM is posed to redesign a new era of food. With this technology, we begin to create foods that meet different criteria such as taste, texture, and high nutritional content. Customizing food facilitates the introduction of a particular food, meeting the needs, tastes, preferences, and eating patterns of different audiences according to their age, gender, occupations, and lifestyles (Lorenz et al. 2022; Mantihal, Kobun, and Lee 2020).

In healthcare, 3D printing facilitates more patient-specific interventions including surgical planning and implant design. Many researchers are studying different bioinks capable of providing a favorable environment for cell proliferation and differentiation. This characteristic is a big step forward for tissue engineering (bones, skin, and organs). With this it will be possible to use the patient's own cells to perform the graft and/or transplant, reducing the risk of rejection. And yet, with 3D printing you can print the structure in the anatomy of each patient.

In addition, it allows the printing of differentiated pharmaceutical forms, such as oral, vaginal, topical, ocular, among others (Applegate et al. 2016; Biranje et al. 2022; Garg et al. 2005; Maver et al. 2018; Pandey et al. 2020; Singh and Jonnalagadda 2021; Wang, Wang, and Xu 2020). With this technology, there is the possibility of printing mimetic environments to the natural, and it plays an integral role in the advancement of tissue engineering and biomedical research (Alam, Varadarajan, and Kumar 2020; Cui et al. 2012; Freeman and Kelly 2017; Hospodiuk et al. 2018). As 3D printing continues to become more sophisticated it is likely to have a major influence on healthcare in the future.

1.3   CUSTOMIZATION

Customization, in which the product is adjusted according to the preferences and anatomy of the consumer and/or patient, is something that has been adopted by some companies (Guo, Choi, and Chung 2022). In recent years, the advancement of technology has allowed and improved the customization of products, while also raising concerns about cost, quality of the final product, and its viability in operations.

AM has become promising in industries in all fields, as it enables the customization of various products. The most interesting thing is that AM allows the creation and development of several structures of high complexity and good resolution without the need for a mold. For the customized structure to be printed, first it is necessary to scan what you want to print and with the help of computer-aided design (CAD) software, this image is sliced and then printed in 3D (Uchida and Bruschi 2023).

The AM of pharmaceutical materials allows the 3D printing of anatomically similar structures to the patient, which favors its use in tissue engineering. In many studies, the promise of reducing the rejection of transplanted and/or grafted tissues (bones, skin, and organs) is what draws the most attention to this technology, which justifies its recent advances. For example, a patient with multiple fractures in the femur, which is a large bone, may have his bone transplanted and 3D printed with the same structure as a natural bone and anatomically similar to that of the patient's.

AM allows the printing of complex structures, therefore the interior of the bioprinted bone has channels and trabeculae, providing a favorable environment for cell proliferation and differentiation, and, thus, bone regeneration. The most interesting thing is that the wide range of printer types allows the choice of an ideal printer that will not damage the cells used.

The same goes for bioprinted artificial skins. In addition to being used for biological tests in research and thus reducing the use of animals, there is the possibility of printing skin for grafts with blood vessels and other structures using the patient's own cells. The 3D printing of these artificial skins can provide a mimetic environment and facilitate the exchange of oxygen with the external environment. Unlike an autograft, with 3D printing there is no need to remove skin from another region of the body, reducing the risk of infections and scarring. As a result, bioprinted skin brings greater biological safety to patients and does not affect their self-esteem, as it does not leave scars. In addition to using the patients' own cells, there is the possibility of adding growth factors and/or other components that will improve the healing process.

Imagine the possibility of printing an organ and thus avoiding waiting for a donor! And additionally, reducing the risk of suffering rejection of that transplanted organ! A dream, isn't it? We are happy to say that this reality is not too far off. The use of the ideal bioink, (non-toxic, biodegradable, and favoring cell proliferation and differentiation) along with the correct 3D bioprinter, and the patient's own cells, will make this dream a reality. The positive point of AM is that this organ will be printed in the same anatomical format as the patient's with the same blood vessels, size, and volume as it has the patient's own cells, the level of rejection is very low. It is not just in the biomedical area that we see the marvel of AM. A treatment focused on the patient's needs and well-being is what everyone wants.

3D printing, in the pharmaceutical area, has drawn attention for providing customization in medication administration. In addition, they offer a personalized treatment in the ideal dosage and size with customized modified release profiles. This makes it much easier for patients of any age to adhere to treatment and reduces incorrect medication dosage.

The pharmaceutical industry makes use of this technology to develop devices that will carry the drug to the desired location. With that in mind, studies like vaginal chips for hormone release; magnetic structures; microneedles to facilitate drug penetration; biofilms for the treatment of various diseases; controlled-release capsules; among others, have been carried out to provide the patient with a more individualized treatment, respecting the correct dosage and preventing overdose (Ajiteru et al. 2021; Dhwaj et al. 2022; Farias et al. 2018; Ibañez et al. 2021; Lantean et al. 2021; Luzuriaga et al. 2018; Shin and Hyun 2021).

In addition, the pharmaceutical dosage form can be printed in the desired format, respecting the patient's anatomy and, in the case of a patient who uses several medications, there is the possibility of printing them in different formats and colors, which can ensure that the patient does not take the medicine in the wrong way. This new form of drug delivery enables greater adherence to therapy in pediatric patients due to the possibility of printing ludic structures.

1.4 ADVANTAGES OVER TRADITIONAL MEDICINES

Unlike traditional medicine, where the medicine is ready and manufactured by identical batches, AM allows printing of a medicine that will meet the needs of the individual and is much more versatile than a conventional treatment (Figure 1.2). Considering that anatomically we are similar and physiologically we can be different from others, we can assume that we are not all the same. Bearing this in mind, we know that everyone has a different pharmacological need than the other, therefore, a drug treatment for one individual differs from the other. Often, when the patient complains that the medication does not work, the problem may lie in the subtherapeutic dosage. And then, the dosage is increased leading to an overdose. The impossibility of providing individualized treatment using traditional treatment results in many pharmacological drawbacks.

Precision and individualization would reduce treatment error. Also, it would reduce waste. Who never finished a drug treatment and ended up with a bunch of pills left? Even with the correct disposal of the medicine, the by-product is discarded inactivated, but it still pollutes nature.

It is known that cases of microbial resistance are related to the exaggerated use of antibiotics, even in a treatment with medical supervision. When using 3D printing medicines, the dose format and size are optimized, consequently the medicine and its material are also optimized, reducing waste from it and the entire production process.

3D PRINTING

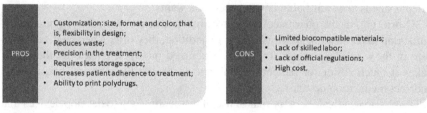

TRADITIONAL TREATMENT

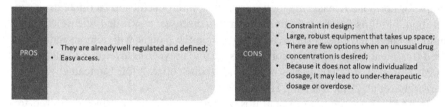

FIGURE 1.2 Pros and cons of traditional treatment and treatment using 3D printing.

3D printed drugs came to reduce these disadvantages of traditional treatment. Offering an individualized and customized treatment to the patient will increase their adherence to the treatment and still improve the treatment. In elderly patients, who usually take several medications, with 3D printing medications can be printed in different formats and colors, which will facilitate the patient's daily life ensuring that the patient does not confuse the medications. In the case of children who have difficulty swallowing a medication, printing a more playful pharmaceutical form will facilitate their adherence.

So far, we have reported on oral medications, but what about topical medications? We start from the same assumption. In a wound, conventional treatment is usually carried out with compresses made of cotton, adhesive bandages, and plasters, but this type of treatment can worsen the wound and impair the healing process by not keeping the microenvironment moist, by preventing the exchange of oxygen with the external environment and can increase the risk of infection. Not to mention that when removing a bandage, for example, if not done carefully, the part that has already started the healing process can open again. With 3D bioprinting of biofilms all these disadvantages are overcome. Due to the high resolution of the 3D bioprinter, these biofilms can be printed with small holes that will facilitate gas exchange and are able to keep the microenvironment moist (Uchida and Bruschi 2023).

Because the bioink is biodegradable, there is no need to remove the biofilm from the wound and what will ensure the customization of the treatment is that these biofilms can be printed in any size and format according to the size of the patient's wound.

The interesting thing is that 3D printing of drugs is eco-friendly, reducing the amount of time, drugs, and inert products that are wasted. In addition, printers do not require a very spacious environment, despite the need for skilled labor. To work with

3D printers, it is necessary to be familiar with slicing and printing software, but it is not difficult, basic training already overcomes this disadvantage.

Unlike traditional treatment, where everything is already consolidated; to use 3D bioprinting, it is essential to choose the correct bioink and your choice will depend on the type of 3D bioprinter and the purpose of the bioprinted material. It is necessary that the bioink is biodegradable, non-toxic, and biocompatible; however, the choice of biopolymer to be used will depend on the type of treatment. That is, the biopolymer that is used to manufacture a 3D bone is different from a biopolymer that is used to print an artificial skin. Although the traditional treatment is consolidated, this does not prevent the use of 3D bioprinted materials, it is enough to have prior knowledge of the ideal bioink for each printer and the purpose.

This shows us that 3D bioprinting has dominant advantages over conventional treatment, always aiming at the best patient care. As with any other type of treatment, challenges must be faced. We will discuss these challenges in the next section.

1.5 ADDITIVE MANUFACTURING CHALLENGES

AM showed effectiveness in its development and applicability in several industrial areas. However, 3D printing presents some limitations and challenges that need to be overcome. The way the printed part is obtained affects surface accuracy, height, and volume. From this, we started the topic with the first challenge to be faced, which is the presence of people specialized in 3D printing in the printed material development group.

The presence of specialized and qualified people avoids the risk of waste and poorly designed structures, thus reducing costs. Having knowledge about the types of printers and knowing how to handle the software and the type of material that can be printed on each type of printer, in addition to reducing costs, also reduces time during the development of a new DDS, for example. In the case of the pharmaceutical industry, geometric characteristics will influence the release of the drug in the desired location. As we can see, the presence of trained personnel is essential and with this, other challenges are already solved, such as producing a structure according to the patient's preferences and needs, as well as offering a short delivery time for personalized material and overcoming the complexity of the products (Palo et al. 2017; Uchida and Bruschi 2023).

Another challenge to be faced is the limited variety of polymers and waxes that can be used for 3D printing in healthcare. There are many types of printers that can be used in the pharmaceutical and biomedical industry, each with its own particularities (see Chapter 2); however, many of these inks or filaments are not intended for application in the healthcare area, which is the reason research has been carried out for the development of more biodegradable, biocompatibility, and non-toxic materials. Some natural polymers from proteins, such as collagen gelatin, have shown promise for obtaining inks for 3D printing, due to their good biological response. However, more studies must be conducted to standardize the viscoelasticity of these inks, which is why understanding the understanding the rheology of printing ink is important.

The lack of laws and regulations is another challenge to be faced. 3D printed materials appear to be very promising in many different industries. However, the lack of supervision and regulations, as with traditional medicines on the market, makes their spread difficult.

When aiming to introduce AM into the market, the FDA launched a booklet with technical considerations on the topic (Food and Drug Administration 2017). This guide is a starting point on the technical considerations of 3D printers. Therefore, it is important to highlight that resolutions involving the introduction of AM in the healthcare market must take into account regulatory considerations that guarantee quality control of printed materials at the beginning of development to the final product, in order to offer the patient the best possible treatment, with safety, effectiveness, and stability.

In the following chapters, 3D printing and its state of the art capacities will be discussed, as well as its application for obtaining new drug delivery systems with bioadhesive properties.

REFERENCES

Ajiteru, O., K. Y. Choi, T. H. Lim, D. Y. Kim, H. Hong, Y. J. Lee, J. S. Lee, et al. 2021. "A Digital Light Processing 3D Printed Magnetic Bioreactor System Using Silk Magnetic Bioink." *Biofabrication* 13 (3): 034102.

Alam, F., K. M. Varadarajan, and S. Kumar. 2020. "3D Printed Polylactic Acid Nanocomposite Scaffolds for Tissue Engineering Applications." *Polymer Testing* 81: 106203.

Albanna, M., K. W. Binder, S. V. Murphy, J. Kim, S. A. Qasem, W. Zhao, J. Tan, et al. 2019. "In Situ Bioprinting of Autologous Skin Cells Accelerates Wound Healing of Extensive Excisional Full-Thickness Wounds." *Scientific Reports* 9 (1): 1–15. https://doi.org/10.1038/s41598-018-38366-w.

Applegate, M. B., B. P. Partlow, J. Coburn, B. Marelli, C. Pirie, R. Pineda, D. L. Kaplan, and F. G. Omenetto. 2016. "Photocrosslinking of Silk Fibroin Using Riboflavin for Ocular Prostheses." *Advanced Materials* 28 (12): 2417–20. Accessed March 28, 2023. https://doi.org/10.1002/ADMA.201504527.

Biranje, S. S., J. Sun, L. Cheng, Y. Cheng, Y. Shi, S. Yu, H. Jiao, et al. 2022. "Development of Cellulose Nanofibril/Casein-Based 3D Composite Hemostasis Scaffold for Potential Wound-Healing Application." *ACS Applied Materials and Interfaces* 14 (3): 3792–808.

Choi, K. Y., O. Ajiteru, H. Hong, Y. J. Suh, M. T. Sultan, H. Lee, J. S. Lee, et al. 2023. "A Digital Light Processing 3D-Printed Artificial Skin Model and Full-Thickness Wound Models Using Silk Fibroin Bioink." *Acta Biomaterialia* S1742–7061 (23): 002349.

Cordeiro, A. S., I. A. Tekko, M. H. Jomaa, L. Vora, E. McAlister, F. Volpe-Zanutto, M. Nethery, et al. 2020. "Two-Photon Polymerisation 3D Printing of Microneedle Array Templates with Versatile Designs: Application in the Development of Polymeric Drug Delivery Systems." *Pharmaceutical Research* 37 (9): 1–15. Accessed June 4, 2023. https://doi.org/10.1007/S11095-020-02887-9/FIGURES/9.

Cui, X., T. Boland, D. D.D'Lima, and M. K. Lotz. 2012. "Thermal Inkjet Printing in Tissue Engineering and Regenerative Medicine." *Recent Patents on Drug Delivery & Formulation* 6 (2): 149–55. Accessed June 4, 2023. https://doi.org/10.2174/187221112800672949.

Dhwaj, A., N. Roy, A. Jaiswar, A. Prabhakar, and D. Verma. 2022. "3D-Printed Impedance Micropump for Continuous Perfusion of the Sample and Nutrient Medium Integrated with a Liver-On-Chip Prototype." *ACS Omega* 7 (45): 40900–910. Accessed April 11, 2023. https://doi.org/10.1021/ACSOMEGA.2C03818/ASSET/IMAGES/LARGE/AO2C03818_0013.JPEG.

Farias, C., R. Lyman, C. Hemingway, H. Chau, A. Mahacek, E. Bouzos, and M. Mobed-Miremadi. 2018. "Three-Dimensional (3D) Printed Microneedles for Microencapsulated Cell Extrusion." *Bioengineering* 5 (3): 59. https://doi.org/10.3390/BIOENGINEERING5030059.

Food and Drug Administration. 2017. "Technical Considerations for Additive Manufactured Medical Devices:Guidance for Industry and Food and Drug Administration Staff Document." FDA. 2017. Accessed October 4, 2022. https://www.fda.gov/media/97633/download.

Freeman, F. E., and D. J. Kelly. 2017. "Tuning Alginate Bioink Stiffness and Composition for Controlled Growth Factor Delivery and to Spatially Direct MSC Fate within Bioprinted Tissues." *Scientific Reports* 7: 1–12.

Garg, S., K. Vermani, A. Garg, R. A. Anderson, W. B. Rencher, and L. J. D. Zaneveld. 2005. "Development and Characterization of Bioadhesive Vaginal Films of Sodium Polystyrene Sulfonate (PSS), a Novel Contraceptive Antimicrobial Agent." *Pharmaceutical Research* 22 (4): 584–95.

Gokhare, V. G., D. N. Raut, and D. K. Shinde. 2017. "A Review Paper on 3D-Printing Aspects and Various Processes Used in the 3D-Printing." *International Journal Os Engineering Research & Technology* 6 (6): 953–58. Accessed May 25, 2023. www.ijert.org.

Guo, S., T. M. Choi, and S. H. Chung. 2022. "Self-Design Fun: Should 3D Printing Be Employed in Mass Customization Operations?" *European Journal of Operational Research* 299 (3): 883–97. Accessed May 27, 2023. https://doi.org/10.1016/J.EJOR.2021.07.009.

Hager, I., A. Golonka, and R. Putanowicz. 2016. "3D Printing of Buildings and Building Components as the Future of Sustainable Construction?" *Procedia Engineering* 151: 292–99. Accessed May 25, 2023. https://doi.org/10.1016/J.PROENG.2016.07.357.

Han, Z., S. Liu, K. Qiu, J. Liu, R. Zou, Y. Wang, J. Zhao, F. Liu, Y. Wang, and L. Li. 2023. "The Enhanced ZrO2 Produced by DLP via a Reliable Plasticizer and Its Dental Application." *Journal of the Mechanical Behavior of Biomedical Materials* 141: 105751.

Hospodiuk, M., K. K. Moncal, M. Dey, and I. T. Ozbolat. 2018. "Extrusion-Based Biofabrication in Tissue Engineering and Regenerative Medicine." *3D Printing and Biofabrication*, 255–81. https://doi.org/10.1007/978-3-319-45444-3_10.

Ibañez, R. I. R., R. J. F. C. Do Amaral, R. L. Reis, A. P. Marques, C. M. Murphy, and F. J. O'brien. 2021. "3D-Printed Gelatin Methacrylate Scaffolds with Controlled Architecture and Stiffness Modulate the Fibroblast Phenotype towards Dermal Regeneration." *Polymers* 13 (15): 2515.

Koide, M., K. Osaki, J. Konishi, K. Oyamada, T. Katakura, A. Takahashi, and K. Yoshizato. 1993. "A New Type of Biomaterial for Artificial Skin: Dehydrothermally Cross-Linked Composites of Fibrillar and Denatured Collagens." *Journal of Biomedical Materials Research* 27 (1): 79–87.

Lantean, S., I. Roppolo, M. Sangermano, M. Hayoun, H. Dammak, and G. Rizza. 2021. "Programming the Microstructure of Magnetic Nanocomposites in DLP 3D Printing." *Additive Manufacturing* 47: 102343.

Li, J., and H. Tanaka. 2018. "Rapid Customization System for 3D-Printed Splint Using Programmable Modeling Technique – a Practical Approach." *3D Printing in Medicine* 4 (1): 1–21. Accessed May 27, 2023. https://doi.org/10.1186/S41205-018-0027-6.

Li, X., B. Liu, B. Pei, J. Chen, D. Zhou, J. Peng, X. Zhang, W. Jia, and T. Xu. 2020. "Inkjet Bioprinting of Biomaterials." *Chemical Reviews* 120 (19): 10793–833. https://doi.org /10.1021/ACS.CHEMREV.0C00008/ASSET/IMAGES/MEDIUM/CR0C00008_0029 .GIF.

Liu, Z., H. Liang, T. Shi, D. Xie, R. Chen, X. Han, L. Shen, C. Wang, and Z. Tian. 2019. "Additive Manufacturing of Hydroxyapatite Bone Scaffolds via Digital Light Processing and in Vitro Compatibility." *Ceramics International* 45 (8): 11079–86.

Lorenz, T., M. M. Iskandar, V. Baeghbali, M. O. Ngadi, and S. Kubow. 2022. "3D Food Printing Applications Related to Dysphagia: A Narrative Review." *Foods* 11 (12).

Luzuriaga, M. A., D. R. Berry, J. C. Reagan, R. A. Smaldone, and J. J. Gassensmith. 2018. "Biodegradable 3D Printed Polymer Microneedles for Transdermal Drug Delivery." *Lab on a Chip* 18 (8): 1223–30. https://doi.org/10.1039/C8LC00098K.

Mantihal, S., R. Kobun, and B. B. Lee. 2020. "3D Food Printing of as the New Way of Preparing Food: A Review." *International Journal of Gastronomy and Food Science* 22 (December): 100260. Accessed June 1, 2022. https://doi.org/10.1016/J.IJGFS.2020 .100260.

Maver, T., D. M. Smrke, M. Kurečič, L. Gradišnik, U. Maver, and K. S. Kleinschek. 2018. "Combining 3D Printing and Electrospinning for Preparation of Pain-Relieving Wound-Dressing Materials." *Journal of Sol-Gel Science and Technology* 88 (1): 33–48. https://doi.org/10.1007/S10971-018-4630-1.

Palo, M., J. Holländer, J. Suominen, J. Yliruusi, and N. Sandler. 2017. "3D Printed Drug Delivery Devices: Perspectives and Technical Challenges." *Expert Review of Medical Devices* 14 (9): 685–96. Accessed October 5, 2023. https://www.tandfonline.com/doi/ abs/10.1080/17434440.2017.1363647.

Pandey, M., H. Choudhury, J. L. C. Fern, A. T. K. Kee, J. Kou, J. L. J. Jing, H. C. Her, et al. 2020. "3D Printing for Oral Drug Delivery: A New Tool to Customize Drug Delivery." *Drug Delivery and Translational Research* 10 (4): 986–1001. https://doi.org/10.1007/ S13346-020-00737-0.

Prashar, G., H. Vasudev, and D. Bhuddhi. 2022. "Additive Manufacturing: Expanding 3D Printing Horizon in Industry 4.0." *International Journal on Interactive Design and Manufacturing*, 1–15. Accessed May 25, 2023. https://doi.org/10.1007/S12008-022 -00956-4/FIGURES/9.

Rajput, M., P. Mondal, P. Yadav, and K. Chatterjee. 2022. "Light-Based 3D Bioprinting of Bone Tissue Scaffolds with Tunable Mechanical Properties and Architecture from Photocurable Silk Fibroin." *International Journal of Biological Macromolecules* 202: 644–56.

Rando, P., and M. Ramaioli. 2021. "Food 3D Printing: Effect of Heat Transfer on Print Stability of Chocolate." *Journal of Food Engineering* 294: 110415. Accessed May 31, 2023. https://doi.org/10.1016/J.JFOODENG.2020.110415.

Shin, D., and J. Hyun. 2021. "Silk Fibroin Microneedles Fabricated by Digital Light Processing 3D Printing." *Journal of Industrial and Engineering Chemistry* 95: 126–33.

Singh, M., and S. Jonnalagadda. 2021. "Design and Characterization of 3D Printed, Neomycin-Eluting Poly-L-Lactide Mats for Wound-Healing Applications." *Journal of Materials Science. Materials in Medicine* 32 (4): 44.

Uchida, D. T., and M. L. Bruschi. 2023. "3D Printing as a Technological Strategy for the Personalized Treatment of Wound Healing." *AAPS PharmSciTech* 24 (1): 1–25.

Wang, J., A. Goyanes, S. Gaisford, and A. W. Basit. 2016. "Stereolithographic (SLA) 3D Printing of Oral Modified-Release Dosage Forms." *International Journal of Pharmaceutics* 503 (1–2): 207–12. Accessed April 1, 2023. https://pubmed.ncbi.nlm .nih.gov/26976500/.

Wang, X., Q. Wang, and C. Xu. 2020. "Nanocellulose-Based Inks for 3d Bioprinting: Key Aspects in Research Development and Challenging Perspectives in Applications—a Mini Review." *Bioengineering* 7 (2): 40.

Wang, Y., S. Chen, H. Liang, Y. Liu, J. Bai, and M. Wang. 2022. "Digital Light Processing (DLP) of Nano Biphasic Calcium Phosphate Bioceramic for Making Bone Tissue Engineering Scaffolds." *Ceramics International* 48 (19): 27681–92.

Wohlers, T., and T. Gornet. 2016. "History of Additive Manufacturing." *Wohlers Report*, 1–38.

Yang, F., M. Zhang, B. Bhandari, and Y. Liu. 2018. "Investigation on Lemon Juice Gel as Food Material for 3D Printing and Optimization of Printing Parameters." *LWT* 87: 67–76. Accessed May 31, 2023. https://doi.org/10.1016/J.LWT.2017.08.054.

Zheng, C., X. Liu, X. Luo, M. Zheng, X. Wang, W. Dan, and H. Jiang. 2019. "Development of a Novel Bio-Inspired 'Cotton-like' Collagen Aggregate/Chitin Based Biomaterial with a Biomimetic 3D Microstructure for Efficient Hemostasis and Tissue Repair." *Journal of Materials Chemistry B* 7 (46): 7338–50.

2 Types of 3D Printers in Topical and Mucosal Applications

2.1 DESIGN FOR ADDITIVE MANUFACTURING

We believe that most people who are going to start 3D printing ask themselves how the structure that they want to print will be printed. While for some this is clear, for others it is not. For this reason, let us clarify how the 3D and/or 4D printing process unfolds.

Due to AM's ability to print complex structures, its use has been enchanting professionals from various areas. First, it is necessary to know the printer that will be used, as well as the type of bioink that will be used by it. In order to print complex structures, specific software is needed that can take an image and print it layer by layer with high resolution, respecting both the internal and external structure.

During the 3D printing process, volumetric pixels, known as voxels, are deposited, come together, and transform into the desired object (Thompson et al. 2016). The shape and size of each voxel and the binding strength between them are determined according to the type of bioink, the type of printer, the printer resolution, the presence, or absence, of light beams, and the size of the printing platform.

The use of computer-aided design (CAD) is fundamental for creation of the desired design. CAD is a software that assists in design modeling, analysis, review, and documentation (Hunde and Woldeyohannes 2022). The desired design must be created using CAD following the appropriate dimensions, and afterwards, the file must be saved as a CAD file. This file will contain all the information on how the 3D printer should proceed. It is in this file that the amount of material that will be deposited is determined (Figure 2.1).

The software has some pre-developed formats, but if you need a more customized 3D printed structure (for example, organs, bones, teeth, among others) it is necessary to have the anatomical image of the patient at hand. To acquire the image, processes such as scanning, tomography, radiography, or ultrasonography must be used (Dadoo et al. 2021; Buonamici et al. 2020; Hunde and Woldeyohannes 2022; Reighard et al. 2021). From the image, the customized structure is modeled in a CAD environment to be 3D printed. However, the CAD modeling procedure requires the skill of an expert modeler.

Customized drug delivery systems can provide an improved solution for accurate dosing, controlled release, and minimally invasive drug delivery. As mentioned,

DOI: 10.1201/9781003442363-2

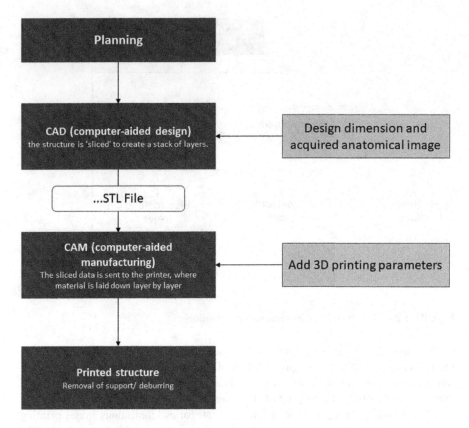

FIGURE 2.1   Flowchart of planning process until obtaining printed material.

there are several types of 3D printers, each with its specificities, particularities, and purposes. Knowing them is the key to adapting and succeeding in 3D printing. Next, the main 3D printers for the pharmaceutical area will be discussed.

2.2   INKJET-BASED PRINTING SYSTEMS

Inkjet-based bioprinting is based on the fabrication of structures using thermal or piezoelectric technology. This technology deposits droplets of low viscosity bioinks on a nano and/or micro scale onto a printing tray. This bioink is inside an inkjet head, the drops of bioinks can be ejected and fixed on substrates on a non-contact surface (X. Li et al. 2020; Evans et al. 2021; Scoutaris, Ross, and Douroumis 2016).

Inkjet-based bioprinting allows the deposition of droplets of a binder bioink on a layer of powder, resulting in the droplet adhering to the powder and forming the desired 3D format (Rowe et al. 2000). The first 3D printed tablet approved by the Food and Drug Administration (FDA), Spritam®, was developed using this 3D printing technology.

This technology has drawn the attention of researchers because it is a method that does not have much contact with the bioink at the time of printing and the feature

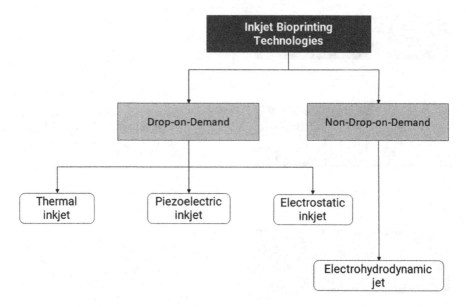

FIGURE 2.2   Flowchart of inkjet bioprinting technologies.

of drop on demand facilitates the standardization of bioinks and avoids wastage of bioink. The size of the droplet produced by 3D inkjet printing is measured in picoliters with the diameter of the printing nozzle approximately 50 μm, a size similar to that of cells, enabling the printing of structures containing cells (X. Li et al. 2020).

Inkjet-based printing is divided into two categories: continuous inkjet printing (non-drop-on-demand) and drop-on-demand inkjet printing (Figure 2.2). Unlike continuous inkjet printing, the drop-on-demand inkjet nozzle produces drops only when the eject signal is reached (X. Li et al. 2020; Scoutaris, Ross, and Douroumis 2016).

2.2.1 Thermal Inkjet

In this technology, the bioink is ejected when heat bubbles are generated by a thermal actuator (heating the bioink for several microseconds). These bubbles squeeze the bioink and form the drop (Figure 2.3). This heating of the thermal actuator can reach 250 to 350 °C; however, as this heating occurs for several microseconds, the temperature of the bioink reaches about 4–10 °C above room temperature (Cui et al. 2012; P. Kumar, Ebbens, and Zhao 2021; Mallinson, McBain, and Brown 2023). Although this heating leads to cell death, most cells remain alive. Some manuscripts show that cell viability after printing is 90%, which is a reasonable and favorable result for printing structures containing cells (Cui et al. 2012; P. Kumar, Ebbens, and Zhao 2021; T. Xu et al. 2013).

Printed-based Inkjet Systems

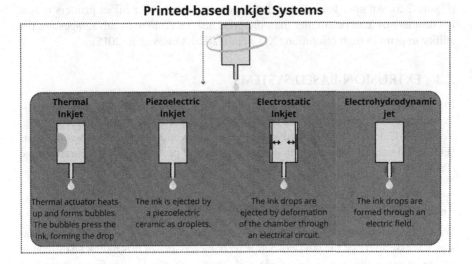

FIGURE 2.3 Schematic representation of 3D printers using the printed-based inkjet systems.

2.2.2 PIEZOELECTRIC INKJET

In a piezoelectric inkjet printer, bioink is ejected by a piezoelectric ceramic as droplets (Figure 2.3). The piezoelectric actuator receives a voltage pulse that generates a deformation in the chamber wall, changing the volume of the bioink, and resulting in the ejection of the drop (bioink). The printhead diameter is 18 to 120 μm and the droplet diameter is between 50 to 100 μm (Boehm et al. 2014; Liang et al. 2022; Wijshoff 2010). The heads of this 3D printer are interchangeable and easy to clean. As heating is not applied in this technology, cell damage caused by increased temperature does not occur (X. Li et al. 2020). However, cell viability using this technology ranges from 70 to95%. Cellular damage caused by the piezoelectric inkjet printer can occur due to pressure, shear, and/or sonication during the ejection process (Gudapati, Dey, and Ozbolat 2016).

2.2.3 ELECTROSTATIC INKJET

During its printing process, the bioink is squeezed by the deformation of the chamber wall, the chamber increases in size and is filled with the bioink (Figure 2.3). When the electrical circuit is disconnected, this chamber returns to its original size and it is at that moment that the drops of bioink are ejected (X. Li et al. 2020).

2.2.4 ELECTROHYDRODYNAMIC JET

With this technology, the bioink drops are formed through an electric field unlike other technologies that squeeze the ink with thermal energy or chamber deformation

(Figure 2.3). Another feature that differentiates it from other inkjet printers is that the droplet size can be smaller than the print nozzle. Among its advantages are the ability to print in high resolution (X. Li et al. 2020; Onses et al. 2015).

2.3 EXTRUSION-BASED SYSTEMS

In this type of 3D printing, the material to be printed is extruded by controlling the xy movement of the extruder and the z position (height) of the build platform (Peng, Vogt, and Cakmak 2018). Extrusion-based systems are divided into two methods (Figure 2.4): fused deposition modeling (FDM) and pressure-assisted microsyringe (PAM).

2.3.1 Pressure-Assisted Microsyringe (PAM)

With PAM printing both liquid and semi-solid materials can be printed. For this reason, it is essential that the physicochemical characteristics of this bioink be evaluated before printing the material (Uchida and Bruschi 2023). Unlike fused deposition modeling (FDM), which we will see in the next section, the PAM technique works at room temperature, which is why understanding the rheology of the material is essential. This technique requires that the bioink to solidify at some point and this semi-solid property must be maintained during the 3D printing of the desired structure without collapsing (El Aita, Breitkreutz, and Quodbach 2019).

The possibility of intercalating two printing nozzles allows the printing of different polymers, generally immiscible, and allows the printing of different active pharmaceutical ingredients (APIs) (El Aita, Breitkreutz, and Quodbach 2019; Elbadawi et al. 2021). Bioink extrusion through the needle occurs when pressure (pneumatic, piston, screw) is applied to the printing syringe (Figure 2.4). The magnitude of the

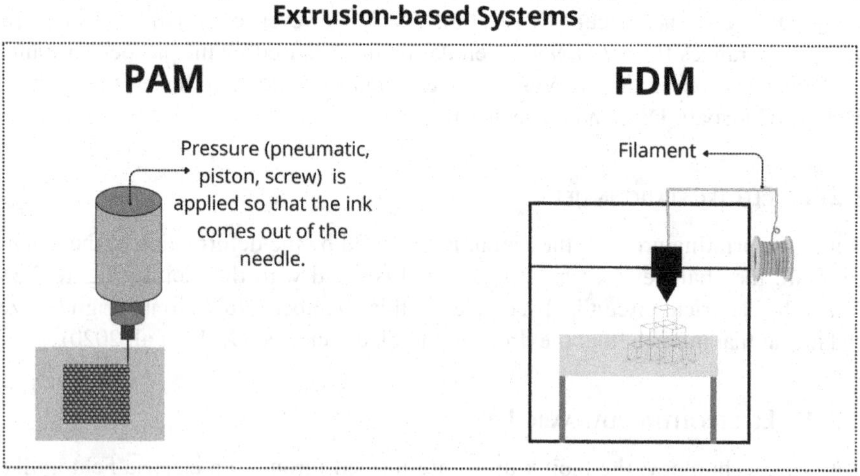

Extrusion-based Systems

FIGURE 2.4 Schematic representation of 3D printers using extrusion-based systems.

applied pressure depends on the rheological behavior of the material, the diameter of the needle, and the shape of the desired structure. Knowing this, the success of PAM printing is dependent on the applied pressure, the diameter of the needle, the extrusion speed, the size and shape of the structure to be printed, and the type of bioink used (Mohammed et al. 2021).

2.3.2 FUSED FILAMENT FABRICATION

Among 3D printers, FDM has the lowest costs and is easiest to handle. The nozzle of the printer heats and melts the thermoplastic filament that is extruded from the syringe needle. The extruded material is deposited layer by layer on a surface. As soon as it leaves the printer nozzle the filament is solidified, forming the desired structure (Figure 2.4) (Dezaki et al. 2021; Goyanes et al. 2015; Hıra et al. 2022; Shaqour et al. 2021).

3D printer using FDM enables the printing of tablets with adequate mechanical strength and its flexibility allows the preparation of pharmaceutical forms with modified release profiles, by varying the density, geometry, and/or arrangement of the printed structure (Eleftheriadis et al. 2020; Fuenmayor et al. 2019; Goyanes et al. 2015). Due to the elevated temperature at the printer's nozzle, this technology only allows the printing of thermostable APIs.

In addition to oral forms, FDM printing enables the printing of scaffolds that favor cell proliferation and devices that enable wound healing (Domínguez-Robles et al. 2019; Intini et al. 2018; Luzuriaga et al. 2018). In this way, there are few biocompatible filaments; however, studies have been conducted aimed at developing a biocompatible, non-toxic filament that provides an environment conducive to cell proliferation. Manufactured filaments with these characteristics and based on poly(lactic acid) (PLA) include polyethylene terephthalate glycol (PETG), poly(ethylene glycol) (PEG), 316L stainless steel powder, among others (Brounstein, Yeager, and Labouriau 2021; Sadaf, Bragaglia, and Nanni 2021; Straker et al. 2023; Vanaei et al. 2020).

2.4 LIGHT-BASED SYSTEM

This technique enables the best printing resolution. The technique consists of obtaining the printed structure through the process of localized photopolymerization, which precisely focuses a beam of light on a photopolymerizable resin that transforms a liquid polymer into a solid structure (Elkhoury, Zuazola, and Vijayavenkataraman 2023). For resin polymerization to occur, the photopolymerizable bioink must contain photoinitiators, which will initiate the polymerization process (Anandakrishnan et al. 2021; Husar et al. 2014). The following are some laser-based system 3D printers, two-photon polymerization (TPP), SLA, and digital light processing (DLP).

2.4.1 TPP

This 3D printing technology is used to print nano and/or micro scale structures. In TPP 3D printing, ultrashort and ultrafast laser pulses (femtoseconds) are focused on

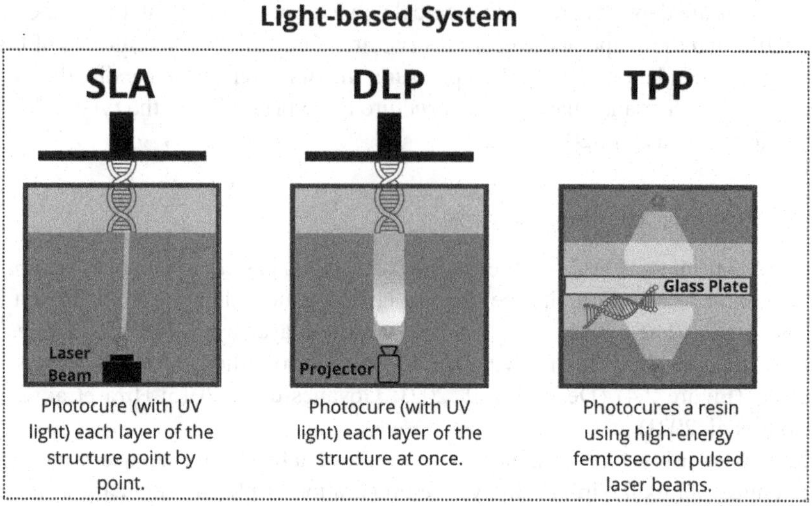

Light-based System

SLA	DLP	TPP
Laser Beam	Projector	Glass Plate
Photocure (with UV light) each layer of the structure point by point.	Photocure (with UV light) each layer of the structure at once.	Photocures a resin using high-energy femtosecond pulsed laser beams.

FIGURE 2.5 Schematic representation of 3D printers using light-based systems and the projection of light in each type of printing: SLA (stereolithography), DLP (digital light processing), and TPP (two-photon polymerization).

a photopolymerizable resin (Figure 2.5). These photons are near infrared (780–820 nm) and the light-curing resin can only be solidified by absorbing two photons simultaneously, which allows printing at nano and micro scales (Cordeiro et al. 2020; Ovsianikov et al. 2006).

Compared with other techniques, this is the one that best controls the geometry of the structure to be printed, with a scalable resolution and minimal maintenance costs (Cordeiro et al. 2020). In terms of resolution, an FDM print has a resolution of 50–200 μm, an SLA print has a resolution of 20 μm, and a TPP has a resolution of 100 nm (Melchels, Feijen, and Grijpma 2010). The design of the device, the porosity, and the density of the material influence the release profile of small molecules, so this technology has been used in the development of new forms of drug delivery and even in tissue engineering (Do et al. 2018; Rad, Prewett, and Davies 2021; Gittard et al. 2010; Xing, Zheng, and Duan 2015).

2.4.2 SLA

This 3D printing technology forms objects layer by layer from photosensitive materials cured using UV radiation, usually at a short wavelength (UV < 400 nm) to initiate the reaction (Figure 2.5) (H. Kumar and Kim 2020). The foundation of this technology is based on the photocuring of the resins, which consists of an exothermic polymerization process through chemical crosslinking reactions.

This reaction begins when a UV light beam is focused on the bioink which causes the curing process to occur (gelling and vitrification) (Domínguez et al. 2010; Ge et al. 2020; Huang, Qin, and Wang 2020; Lange et al. 2000). During gelation, the liquid bioink transitions into a more viscous bioink, in this transition this viscous bioink (gel) turns into a solid material (vitrification).

The main advantage of SLA printing is its versatility, as with this technology it is possible to incorporate drugs into the bioink before printing and the drug is linked and trapped in the photocurable matrices. With SLA, it is possible to manufacture 3D bioprinted oral dosage forms incorporating different drugs in one tablet (Healy et al. 2019; J. Wang et al. 2016; X. Xu et al. 2021). Due to non-heat involvement, ease of preparation of drug-loaded photocurable bioinks, and high resolution these photo-polymerization-based techniques have attracted much interest in the manufacture of solid oral dosage forms and in the printing of thermally unstable drug dosage forms (J. Wang et al., 2016). In addition, due to the high resolution of the printer, several structures can be printed, including biological structures for possible grafts and trans-plants (Anandakrishnan et al. 2021; Farzan et al. 2020; H. Kumar and Kim 2020).

TPP and SLA are 3D printing technologies based on laser scanning; therefore, they are relatively slow, as they locally photopolymerize the bioink point by point (Ge et al. 2020). With digital light processing (DLP), bioprinting occurs faster than with others.

2.4.3 DLP

DLP consists of the projection of UV light (365–405 nm) on a photocurable bioink (Kuang et al. 2019; Mao et al. 2020; Yuan et al. 2019). This UV light is modulated by a digital micromirror device (DMD) chip and the light is projected, curing the bioink layer by layer (Figure 2.5) (Kadry et al. 2019; Y. Li et al. 2021; L. Wang et al. 2019). The DMD consists of a group of micron-sized controllable mirrors that rotate and control the path of the light beam, projecting light onto the photocurable bioink. In this DLP printing technology, the layer is formed in a single exposure and the layer can be scaled, depending on the optical system, to a small size (20–50 μm).

Comparing SLA and DLP printers, DLP printers are more efficient, more flexible, faster, and can be operated in a wider wavelength range. In addition, it allows the use of smaller amounts of photocurable bioink, because the reservoirs (vat) can be cus-tomized (Kadry et al. 2019). This versatility and high resolution of the DLP printer allows the printing of different structures for the biomedical and pharmaceutical area (Geng 2011; Huh et al. 2021; Lantean et al. 2021).

The mild printing conditions and the process without elevated temperature and shearing of the bioink, allows the printing of living tissues, organs, and bones with-out causing cell damage, even favoring cell proliferation (He et al. 2021; Martinez et al. 2019; Preobrazhenskiy et al. 2021; Xie et al. 2022). This feature also allows the printing of thermosensitive drugs, which makes it possible to print oral pharmaceuti-cal drugs such as capsules and tablets (Kadry et al. 2019).

REFERENCES

Agrim Dadoo, Shipra Jain, Apoorva Mowar, Vishal Bansal, and Anshul Trivedi. 2021. "3D Printing Using CAD Technology or 3D Scanners, A Paradigm Shift in Dentistry – A Review." *Article in Journal of International Dental and Medical Research* 1 (2): 35–40. Accessed May 30, 2023. https://www.researchgate.net/publication/370003446.

Aita, I. El, J. Breitkreutz, and J. Quodbach. 2019. "On-Demand Manufacturing of Immediate Release Levetiracetam Tablets Using Pressure-Assisted Microsyringe Printing." *European Journal of Pharmaceutics and Biopharmaceutics* 134: 29–36. Accessed June 4, 2023. https://doi.org/10.1016/J.EJPB.2018.11.008.

Anandakrishnan, N., H. Ye, Z. Guo, Z. Chen, K. I. Mentkowski, J. K. Lang, N. Rajabian, et al. 2021. "Fast Stereolithography Printing of Large-Scale Biocompatible Hydrogel Models." *Advanced Healthcare Materials* 10 (10): 2002103. Accessed June 4, 2023. https://doi.org/10.1002/ADHM.202002103.

Boehm, R. D., P. R. Miller, J. Daniels, S. Stafslien, and R. J. Narayan. 2014. "Inkjet Printing for Pharmaceutical Applications." *Materials Today* 17 (5): 247–52. Accessed June 4, 2023. https://doi.org/10.1016/J.MATTOD.2014.04.027.

Brounstein, Z., C. M. Yeager, and A. Labouriau. 2021. "Development of Antimicrobial PLA Composites for Fused Filament Fabrication." *Polymers* 13 (4): 580. Accessed June 5, 2023. https://doi.org/10.3390/POLYM13040580.

Buonamici, F., R. Furferi, L. Governi, S. Lazzeri, K. S. McGreevy, M. Servi, E. Talanti, F. Uccheddu, and Y. Volpe. 2020. "A Practical Methodology for Computer-Aided Design of Custom 3D Printable Casts for Wrist Fractures." *Visual Computer*, 375–90. Accessed May 30, 2023. https://link.springer.com/article/10.1007/s00371-018-01624-z.

Cordeiro, A. S., I. A. Tekko, M. H. Jomaa, L. Vora, E. McAlister, F. Volpe-Zanutto, M. Nethery, et al. 2020. "Two-Photon Polymerisation 3D Printing of Microneedle Array Templates with Versatile Designs: Application in the Development of Polymeric Drug Delivery Systems." *Pharmaceutical Research* 37 (9): 1–15. Accessed June 4, 2023. https://doi.org/10.1007/S11095-020-02887-9/FIGURES/9.

Cui, X., T. Boland, D. D. D'Lima, and M. K. Lotz. 2012. "Thermal Inkjet Printing in Tissue Engineering and Regenerative Medicine." *Recent Patents on Drug Delivery & Formulation* 6 (2): 149–55. Accessed June 4, 2023. https://doi.org/10.2174/187221112800672949.

Dezaki, M. L., M. K. A. M. Ariffin, A. Serjouei, A. Zolfagharian, S. Hatami, and M. Bodaghi. 2021. "Influence of Infill Patterns Generated by CAD and FDM 3D Printer on Surface Roughness and Tensile Strength Properties." *Applied Sciences 2021* 11 (16): 7272. Accessed May 29, 2023. https://doi.org/10.3390/APP11167272.

Do, A. V., K. S. Worthington, B. A. Tucker, and A. K. Salem. 2018. "Controlled Drug Delivery from 3D Printed Two-Photon Polymerized Poly(Ethylene Glycol) Dimethacrylate Devices." *International Journal of Pharmaceutics* 552 (1–2): 217–24. Accessed June 1, 2023. https://doi.org/10.1016/J.IJPHARM.2018.09.065.

Domínguez, J. C., M. V. Alonso, M. Oliet, and F. Rodríguez. 2010. "Chemorheological Study of the Curing Kinetics of a Phenolic Resol Resin Gelled." *European Polymer Journal* 46 (1): 50–57. Accessed June 4, 2023. https://doi.org/10.1016/J.EURPOLYMJ.2009.09.004.

Domínguez-Robles, J., N. K. Martin, M. L. Fong, S. A. Stewart, N. J. Irwin, M. I. Rial-Hermida, R. F. Donnelly, and E. Larrañeta. 2019. "Antioxidant PLA Composites Containing Lignin for 3D Printing Applications: A Potential Material for Healthcare Applications." *Pharmaceutics* 11 (4): 165.

Elbadawi, M., D. Nikjoo, T. Gustafsson, S. Gaisford, and A. W. Basit. 2021. "Pressure-Assisted Microsyringe 3D Printing of Oral Films Based on Pullulan and Hydroxypropyl Methylcellulose." *International Journal of Pharmaceutics* 595: 120197. Accessed June 4, 2023. https://doi.org/10.1016/J.IJPHARM.2021.120197.

Eleftheriadis, G. K., C. S. Katsiotis, N. Genina, J. Boetker, J. Rantanen, and D. G. Fatouros. 2020. "Manufacturing of Hybrid Drug Delivery Systems by Utilizing the Fused Filament Fabrication (FFF) Technology." *Expert Opinion on Drug Delivery* 17 (8): 1063–68. Accessed June 5, 2023. https://doi.org/10.1080/17425247.2020.1776260.

Elkhoury, K., J. Zuazola, and S. Vijayavenkataraman. 2023. "Bioprinting the Future Using Light: A Review on Photocrosslinking Reactions, Photoreactive Groups, and Photoinitiators." *SLAS Technology*. Accessed June 4, 2023. https://doi.org/10.1016/J.SLAST.2023.02.003.

Evans, S. E., T. Harrington, M. C. Rodriguez Rivero, E. Rognin, T. Tuladhar, and R. Daly. 2021. "2D and 3D Inkjet Printing of Biopharmaceuticals – A Review of Trends and Future Perspectives in Research and Manufacturing." *International Journal of Pharmaceutics* 599: 120443.

Faraji Rad, Z., P. D. Prewett, and G. J. Davies. 2021. "High-Resolution Two-Photon Polymerization: The Most Versatile Technique for the Fabrication of Microneedle Arrays." *Microsystems & Nanoengineering* 7 (1): 1–17. Accessed June 4, 2023. https://doi.org/10.1038/s41378-021-00298-3.

Farzan, A., S. Borandeh, N. Zanjanizadeh Ezazi, S. Lipponen, H. A. Santos, and J. Seppälä. 2020. "3D Scaffolding of Fast Photocurable Polyurethane for Soft Tissue Engineering by Stereolithography: Influence of Materials and Geometry on Growth of Fibroblast Cells." *European Polymer Journal* 139: 109988.

Fuenmayor, E., M. Forde, A. V. Healy, D. M. Devine, J. G. Lyons, C. McConville, and I. Major. 2019. "Comparison of Fused-Filament Fabrication to Direct Compression and Injection Molding in the Manufacture of Oral Tablets." *International Journal of Pharmaceutics* 558: 328–40. Accessed June 5, 2023. https://doi.org/10.1016/J.IJPHARM.2019.01.013.

Ge, Q., Z. Li, Z. Wang, K. Kowsari, W. Zhang, X. He, J. Zhou, and N. X. Fang. 2020. "Projection Micro Stereolithography Based 3D Printing and Its Applications." *International Journal of Extreme Manufacturing* 2 (2): 022004. Accessed June 4, 2023. https://doi.org/10.1088/2631-7990/AB8D9A.

Geng, J. 2011. "DLP-Based Structured Light 3D Imaging Technologies and Applications." *Emerging Digital Micromirror Device Based Systems and Applications III* 7932: 79320B.

Gittard, S. D., A. Ovsianikov, B. N. Chichkov, A. Doraiswamy, and R. J. Narayan. 2010. "Two-Photon Polymerization of Microneedles for Transdermal Drug Delivery." *Expert Opinion on Drug Delivery* 7 (4): 513–33. Accessed June 4, 2023. https://doi.org/10.1517/17425241003628171.

Goyanes, A., A. B. M. Buanz, G. B. Hatton, S. Gaisford, and A. W. Basit. 2015. "3D Printing of Modified-Release Aminosalicylate (4-ASA and 5-ASA) Tablets." *European Journal of Pharmaceutics and Biopharmaceutics* 89: 157–62. Accessed June 4, 2023. https://doi.org/10.1016/J.EJPB.2014.12.003.

Gudapati, H., M. Dey, and I. Ozbolat. 2016. "A Comprehensive Review on Droplet-Based Bioprinting: Past, Present and Future." *Biomaterials* 102: 20–42. Accessed June 4, 2023. https://doi.org/10.1016/J.BIOMATERIALS.2016.06.012.

He, Y., F. Wang, X. Wang, J. Zhang, D. Wang, and X. Huang. 2021. "A Photocurable Hybrid Chitosan/Acrylamide Bioink for DLP Based 3D Bioprinting." *Materials & Design* 202: 109588.

Healy, A. V., E. Fuenmayor, P. Doran, L. M. Geever, C. L. Higginbotham, and J. G. Lyons. 2019. "Additive Manufacturing of Personalized Pharmaceutical Dosage Forms via Stereolithography." *Pharmaceutics* 11 (12): 645. Accessed June 4, 2023. https://doi.org/10.3390/PHARMACEUTICS11120645.

Hıra, O., S. Yücedağ, S. Samankan, Ö. Y. Çiçek, and A. Altınkaynak. 2022. "Numerical and Experimental Analysis of Optimal Nozzle Dimensions for FDM Printers." *Progress in Additive Manufacturing 2021* 7 (5): 823–38.

Huang, J., Q. Qin, and J. Wang. 2020. "A Review of Stereolithography: Processes and Systems." *Processes* 8 (9): 1138. Accessed June 4, 2023. https://doi.org/10.3390/PR8091138.

Huh, J. T., Y. W. Moon, J. Park, A. Atala, J. J. Yoo, and S. J. Lee. 2021. "Combinations of Photoinitiator and UV Absorber for Cell-Based Digital Light Processing (DLP) Bioprinting." *Biofabrication* 13 (3): 034103. Accessed June 4, 2023. https://doi.org/10.1088/1758-5090/ABFD7A.

Husar, B., M. Hatzenbichler, V. Mironov, R. Liska, J. Stampfl, and A. Ovsianikov. 2014. "Photopolymerization-Based Additive Manufacturing for the Development of 3D Porous Scaffolds." In *Biomaterials for Bone Regeneration: Novel Techniques and Applications*, edited by Peter Dubruel and Sandra Van Vlierberghe, 149–201. Woodhead Publishing. Accessed June 4, 2023. https://doi.org/10.1533/9780857098104.2.149.

Intini, C., L. Elviri, J. Cabral, S. Mros, C. Bergonzi, A. Bianchera, L. Flammini, et al. 2018. "3D-Printed Chitosan-Based Scaffolds: An in Vitro Study of Human Skin Cell Growth and an in-Vivo Wound Healing Evaluation in Experimental Diabetes in Rats." *Carbohydrate Polymers* 199: 593–602.

Kadry, H., S. Wadnap, C. Xu, and F. Ahsan. 2019. "Digital Light Processing (DLP) 3D-Printing Technology and Photoreactive Polymers in Fabrication of Modified-Release Tablets." *European Journal of Pharmaceutical Sciences* 135: 60–67.

Kuang, X., J. Wu, K. Chen, Z. Zhao, Z. Ding, F. Hu, D. Fang, and H. J. Qi. 2019. "Grayscale Digital Light Processing 3D Printing for Highly Functionally Graded Materials." *Science Advances* 5 (5). Accessed June 4, 2023. https://doi.org/10.1126/SCIADV.AAV5790/SUPPL_FILE/AAV5790_SM.PDF.

Kumar, H., and K. Kim. 2020. "Stereolithography 3D Bioprinting." In *Methods in Molecular Biology*, edited by J. M. Crook, 2140:93–108. New York: Humana Press Inc. Accessed June 4, 2023. https://doi.org/10.1007/978-1-0716-0520-2_6/COVER.

Kumar, P., S. Ebbens, and X. Zhao. 2021. "Inkjet Printing of Mammalian Cells – Theory and Applications." *Bioprinting* 23: e00157. Accessed June 4, 2023. https://doi.org/10.1016/J.BPRINT.2021.E00157.

Lange, J., N. Altmann, C. T. Kelly, and P. J. Halley. 2000. "Understanding Vitrification during Cure of Epoxy Resins Using Dynamic Scanning Calorimetry and Rheological Techniques." *Polymer* 41 (15): 5949–55. Accessed June 4, 2023. https://doi.org/10.1016/S0032-3861(99)00758-2.

Lantean, S., I. Roppolo, M. Sangermano, M. Hayoun, H. Dammak, and G. Rizza. 2021. "Programming the Microstructure of Magnetic Nanocomposites in DLP 3D Printing." *Additive Manufacturing* 47: 102343.

Li, X., B. Liu, B. Pei, J. Chen, D. Zhou, J. Peng, X. Zhang, W. Jia, and T. Xu. 2020. "Inkjet Bioprinting of Biomaterials." *Chemical Reviews* 120 (19): 10793–833. https://doi.org/10.1021/ACS.CHEMREV.0C00008/ASSET/IMAGES/MEDIUM/CR0C00008_0029.GIF.

Li, Y., Q. Mao, J. Yin, Y. Wang, J. Fu, and Y. Huang. 2021. "Theoretical Prediction and Experimental Validation of the Digital Light Processing (DLP) Working Curve for Photocurable Materials." *Additive Manufacturing* 37: 101716. Accessed June 4, 2023. https://doi.org/10.1016/J.ADDMA.2020.101716.

Liang, J., H. Zeng, L. Qiao, H. Jiang, Q. Ye, Z. Wang, B. Liu, and Z. Fan. 2022. "3D Printed Piezoelectric Wound Dressing with Dual Piezoelectric Response Models for Scar-Prevention Wound Healing." *ACS Applied Materials and Interfaces* 14 (27): 30507–22.

Luzuriaga, M. A., D. R. Berry, J. C. Reagan, R. A. Smaldone, and J. J. Gassensmith. 2018. "Biodegradable 3D Printed Polymer Microneedles for Transdermal Drug Delivery." *Lab on a Chip* 18 (8): 1223–30. https://doi.org/10.1039/C8LC00098K.

Mallinson, S. G., G. D. McBain, and B. R. Brown. 2023. "Conjugate Heat Transfer in Thermal Inkjet Printheads." *Fluids 2023* 8 (3): 88. Accessed June 4, 2023. https://doi.org/10.3390/FLUIDS8030088.

Mao, Q., Y. Wang, Y. Li, S. Juengpanich, W. Li, M. Chen, J. Yin, J. Fu, and X. Cai. 2020. "Fabrication of Liver Microtissue with Liver Decellularized Extracellular Matrix (DECM) Bioink by Digital Light Processing (DLP) Bioprinting." *Materials Science & Engineering. C, Materials for Biological Applications* 109.

Martinez, M. G., A. J. Bullock, S. MacNeil, and I. U. Rehman. 2019. "Characterisation of Structural Changes in Collagen with Raman Spectroscopy." *Applied Spectroscopy Reviews* 54 (6): 509–42. Accessed June 15, 2023. https://doi.org/10.1080/05704928.2018.1506799.

Melchels, F. P. W., J. Feijen, and D. W. Grijpma. 2010. "A Review on Stereolithography and Its Applications in Biomedical Engineering." *Biomaterials* 31 (24): 6121–30. Accessed June 4, 2023. https://doi.org/10.1016/J.BIOMATERIALS.2010.04.050.

Mohammed, A. A., M. S. Algahtani, M. Z. Ahmad, and J. Ahmad. 2021. "Optimization of Semisolid Extrusion (Pressure-Assisted Microsyringe)-Based 3D Printing Process for Advanced Drug Delivery Application." *Annals of 3D Printed Medicine* 2: 100008. Accessed June 4, 2023. https://doi.org/10.1016/J.STLM.2021.100008.

Onses, M. S., E. Sutanto, P. M. Ferreira, A. G. Alleyne, and J. A. Rogers. 2015. "Mechanisms, Capabilities, and Applications of High-Resolution Electrohydrodynamic Jet Printing." *Small* 11 (34): 4237–66. Accessed June 4, 2023. https://doi.org/10.1002/SMLL.201500593.

Ovsianikov, A., S. Passinger, R. Houbertz, and B. N. Chichkov. 2006. "Three Dimensional Material Processing with Femtosecond Lasers." In *Springer Series in Optical Sciences*, edited by Phips C, 129:121–57. Springer Verlag. Accessed June 4, 2023. https://doi.org/10.1007/978-0-387-30453-3_6/COVER.

Peng, F., B. D. Vogt, and M. Cakmak. 2018. "Complex Flow and Temperature History during Melt Extrusion in Material Extrusion Additive Manufacturing." *Additive Manufacturing* 22: 197–206. Accessed June 4, 2023. https://doi.org/10.1016/J.ADDMA.2018.05.015.

Preobrazhenskiy, I. I., A. A. Tikhonov, P. V. Evdokimov, A. V. Shibaev, and V. I. Putlyaev. 2021. "DLP Printing of Hydrogel/Calcium Phosphate Composites for the Treatment of Bone Defects." *Open Ceramics* 6: 100115.

Regassa Hunde, B., and A. Debebe Woldeyohannes. 2022. "Future Prospects of Computer-Aided Design (CAD) – A Review from the Perspective of Artificial Intelligence (AI), Extended Reality, and 3D Printing." *Results in Engineering* 14: 100478.

Reighard, C. L., A. R. Powell, T. Y. Zurawski, D. M. Rooney, C. A. Keilin, and D. A. Zopf. 2021. "Development of a Novel Mandibular Distraction Osteogenesis Simulator Using Computer Aided Design and 3D Printing." *International Journal of Pediatric Otorhinolaryngology* 142: 110616. Accessed May 30, 2023. https://doi.org/10.1016/J.IJPORL.2021.110616.

Rowe, C. W., W. E. Katstra, R. D. Palazzolo, B. Giritlioglu, P. Teung, and M. J. Cima. 2000. "Multimechanism Oral Dosage Forms Fabricated by Three Dimensional Printing™." *Journal of Controlled Release* 66 (1): 11–17. Accessed June 4, 2023. https://doi.org/10.1016/S0168-3659(99)00224-2.

Sadaf, M., M. Bragaglia, and F. Nanni. 2021. "A Simple Route for Additive Manufacturing of 316L Stainless Steel via Fused Filament Fabrication." *Journal of Manufacturing Processes* 67: 141–50. Accessed June 5, 2023. https://doi.org/10.1016/J.JMAPRO.2021 .04.055.

Scoutaris, N., S. Ross, and D. Douroumis. 2016. "Current Trends on Medical and Pharmaceutical Applications of Inkjet Printing Technology." *Pharmaceutical Research* 33 (8): 1799–816.

Shaqour, B., M. Abuabiah, S. Abdel-Fattah, A. Juaidi, R. Abdallah, W. Abuzaina, M. Qarout, B. Verleije, and P. Cos. 2021. "Gaining a Better Understanding of the Extrusion Process in Fused Filament Fabrication 3D Printing: A Review." *International Journal of Advanced Manufacturing Technology* 114: 1279–91. Accessed June 5, 2023. https://doi .org/10.1007/S00170-021-06918-6/FIGURES/1.

Straker, M. A., J. A. Levy, J. M. Stine, V. Borbash, L. A. Beardslee, and R. Ghodssi. 2023. "Freestanding Region-Responsive Bilayer for Functional Packaging of Ingestible Devices." *Microsystems & Nanoengineering* 9 (1): 1–11. Accessed October 8, 2023. https://doi.org/10.1038/s41378-023-00536-w.

Thompson, M. K., G. Moroni, T. Vaneker, G. Fadel, R. I. Campbell, I. Gibson, A. Bernard, et al. 2016. "Design for Additive Manufacturing: Trends, Opportunities, Considerations, and Constraints." *CIRP Annals* 65 (2): 737–60. Accessed May 30, 2023. https://doi.org /10.1016/J.CIRP.2016.05.004.

Uchida, D. T., and M. L. Bruschi. 2023. "3D Printing as a Technological Strategy for the Personalized Treatment of Wound Healing." *AAPS PharmSciTech* 24 (1): 1–25.

Vanaei, H., M. Shirinbayan, M. Deligant, K. Raissi, J. Fitoussi, S. Khelladi, and A. Tcharkhtchi. 2020. "Influence of Process Parameters on Thermal and Mechanical Properties of Polylactic Acid Fabricated by Fused Filament Fabrication." *Polymer Engineering & Science* 60 (8): 1822–31. Accessed June 5, 2023. https://doi.org/10.1002/PEN.25419.

Wang, J., A. Goyanes, S. Gaisford, and A. W. Basit. 2016. "Stereolithographic (SLA) 3D Printing of Oral Modified-Release Dosage Forms." *International Journal of Pharmaceutics* 503 (1–2): 207–12. Accessed June 4, 2023. https://doi.org/10.1016/J .IJPHARM.2016.03.016.

Wang, L., Y. Luo, Z. Yang, W. Dai, X. Liu, J. Yang, B. Lu, and L. Chen. 2019. "Accelerated Refilling Speed in Rapid Stereolithography Based on Nano-Textured Functional Release Film." *Additive Manufacturing* 29: 100791. Accessed June 4, 2023. https://doi .org/10.1016/J.ADDMA.2019.100791.

Wijshoff, H. 2010. "The Dynamics of the Piezo Inkjet Printhead Operation." *Physics Reports* 491 (4–5): 77–177. Accessed June 4, 2023. https://doi.org/10.1016/J.PHYSREP.2010.03 .003.

Xie, X., S. Wu, S. Mou, N. Guo, Z. Wang, and J. Sun. 2022. "Microtissue-Based Bioink as a Chondrocyte Microshelter for DLP Bioprinting." *Advanced Healthcare Materials* 11 (22): e2201877.

Xing, J. F., M. L. Zheng, and X. M. Duan. 2015. "Two-Photon Polymerization Microfabrication of Hydrogels: An Advanced 3D Printing Technology for Tissue Engineering and Drug Delivery." *Chemical Society Reviews* 44 (15): 5031–39. Accessed June 1, 2023. https:// doi.org/10.1039/C5CS00278H.

Xu, T., W. Zhao, J. M. Zhu, M. Z. Albanna, J. J. Yoo, and A. Atala. 2013. "Complex Heterogeneous Tissue Constructs Containing Multiple Cell Types Prepared by Inkjet Printing Technology." *Biomaterials* 34 (1): 130–39. https://doi.org/10.1016/J .BIOMATERIALS.2012.09.035.

Xu, X., A. Goyanes, S. J. Trenfield, L. Diaz-Gomez, C. Alvarez-Lorenzo, S. Gaisford, and A. W. Basit. 2021. "Stereolithography (SLA) 3D Printing of a Bladder Device for Intravesical Drug Delivery." *Materials Science and Engineering C* 120.

Yuan, C., K. Kowsari, S. Panjwani, Z. Chen, D. Wang, B. Zhang, C. J. X. Ng, P. V. Y. Alvarado, and Q. Ge. 2019. "Ultrafast Three-Dimensional Printing of Optically Smooth Microlens Arrays by Oscillation-Assisted Digital Light Processing." *ACS Applied Materials and Interfaces* 11 (43): 40662–68. Accessed June 4, 2023. https://doi.org/10.1021/ACSAMI .9B14692/ASSET/IMAGES/LARGE/AM9B14692_0005.JPEG.

3 Drug Delivery Systems

3.1 CONTROLLED DRUG RELEASE SYSTEMS

3.1.1 ACTIVE PHARMACEUTICAL INGREDIENTS

To start this chapter, let's understand the meaning of active pharmaceutical ingredients (APIs). Basically, APIs are a substance or compound (recognized in the official pharmacopoeia) intended for use in the diagnosis, cure, mitigation, treatment, or prevention of diseases (FDA 2015). In this way, APIs are a term used to refer to the substances contained in a medicine responsible for a pharmacological effect on the body.

The APIs can have different origins and ways of being obtained, such as from natural or synthetic sources. For many years, the use of natural products, such as therapeutic agents, was explored and studied by different populations. In this way, several drugs widely used in everyday life were originally obtained from plants, animals, or microorganisms. However, aiming for a broad production and distribution of these therapeutic agents, optimizing their production was necessary. In this way, the syntheses of these natural therapeutic agents were developed and improved, just as through the synthesis of drugs, complex molecules for the treatment of various diseases were developed.

For the development and design of drug delivery systems, knowledge about the intrinsic properties and characteristics of APIs must be well studied. Each API has physicochemical properties that can influence its absorption in the body and, consequently, its therapeutic action. For example, APIs may have low solubility in water, influencing their absorption in the gastrointestinal environment or may have an unpleasant taste and/or odor, making them difficult to administer orally.

Therefore, a comprehensive understanding of the API present in the release system being designed is extremely important, as it is due to these characteristics that the best system will be developed.

3.1.2 ROUTES OF ADMINISTRATION

According to the treatment or prevention, the target tissue, dose, and physicochemical properties of APIs, a route of administration must be determined. These routes of administration are responsible for introducing the API to the site of action in the body and starting the therapeutic action. There are various routes, such as oral, vaginal, parenteral, topical, etc. (Figure 3.1).

The choice of the most effective route of administration is important for developing controlled drug release systems. The APIs have intrinsic physicochemical

DOI: 10.1201/9781003442363-3

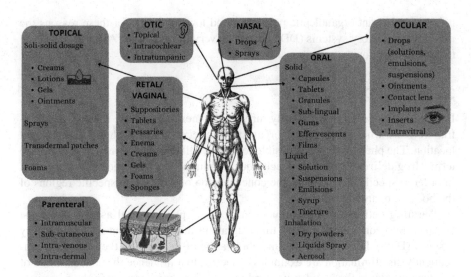

FIGURE 3.1 Possible administration routes for active pharmaceutical ingredients (APIs).

characteristics that can make the treatment complicated, depending on the route they are administered, such as APIs that are poorly soluble in the gastrointestinal environment, for example. Thus, the development of a controlled release system aims to obtain a more comfortable and appropriate administration, helping to improve patient compliance and producing a more appropriate treatment.

The most comfortable, safe, and accessible route is the oral route, making it the most popular among patients. Furthermore, through this route, medications can be self-administered, eliminating the need for trained professionals and a suitable location for administration, unlike the parenteral route, for example. Consequently, most marketed medications are administered via this route. However, the oral route has some disadvantages such as possible interactions with food, the instability of APIs in the pH of gastric fluid, and their low solubility in water, in addition, the presence of unpleasant tastes and/or odors can be a problem.

The intravenous route has rapid action and can be used for medications that need to be administered in large volumes. The intramuscular route also has good absorption, but it can be painful and can cause irritation in the muscles. Therefore, these routes are invasive and require trained professionals and a suitable location.

Therefore, due to the characteristics and physiological factors involved in each route of administration, the development of controlled drug release systems must be designed to optimize their administration and drug performance at the site of action.

The direct use of APIs is very rare and often impractical, since their correct handling and application is very difficult, especially for very potent medicines. Imagine the intravaginal application of an API in the form of crystals or applying an API in the form of a powder into the eyes, it is unfeasible and uncomfortable for the patient; also, this practice can cause local irritation or injuries. Furthermore, many APIs are sensitive to light exposure, and changes in pH, temperature, and humidity, or may present unpleasant organoleptic properties and low solubility, for these reasons the use of drug delivery systems (DDS) becomes very important for API transportation to the site of action.

3.1.3 Drug Delivery Systems

Drugs are introduced into the body through the most appropriate route of administration. Thus, when present in the organism, it is necessary to reach the correct target location. The phenomenon responsible for this is called drug delivery. Therefore, the term "drug delivery" refers to a technique of administering medication to a patient in order to specifically increase the concentration of the drug in specific regions of the body compared to others.

The drug delivery can be influenced by some physiological aspects that must be taken into consideration when thinking about the development of drug delivery systems (DDS). For example, the metabolization of the drug by the body and, consequently, its elimination are examples of factors that influence the concentration of the drug present in the bloodstream and the time it remains present in the organism. Therefore, a drug that is quickly metabolized and excreted requires higher doses of administration in a shorter period, which can cause difficulties in treatment and have low patient adherence.

Also, the route of administration influences the absorption and bioavailability (amount of drug present in the bloodstream) of the drug. For example, there is a bioavailability close to 100% when the parenteral route of administration is used; however, when we think about oral administration, the absorption of the drug can be influenced by several factors such as solubility in the gastrointestinal environment, first pass effect, among others, resulting in lower bioavailability.

Furthermore, from pharmacokinetic studies, it is known that each drug has a toxic concentration, that is, a concentration that, if exceeded, can cause harmful effects on the body, and a subtherapeutic concentration, a minimum concentration that must be introduced to the body to achieve the desired therapeutic effect.

Therefore, a drug administered parenterally can reach a toxic level due to high bioavailability if doses are not administered at a correct interval. Likewise, through oral administration, due to lower bioavailability, the drug can be introduced at a concentration lower than subtherapeutic. Furthermore, due to metabolization and elimination, subsequent doses of the drug may result in a drug concentration outside the therapeutic range (Figure 3.2).

Analyzing the issues addressed above, there are cases where drug delivery must be controlled. For example, a drug administered orally that has its doses administered inappropriately (curve B and C in Figure 3.2) can have its delivery modified so that the entire concentration of the drug remains within the therapeutic range (Figure 3.3).

Modified drug release means that the release of the API is different from the traditional release. Based on this assumption, modified release pharmaceutical forms (MRPFs) are those whose characteristics of time and/or location of drug release are determined to target therapeutic, or convenience objectives not offered

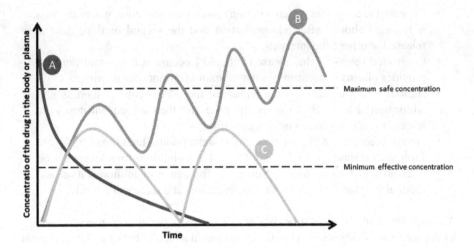

FIGURE 3.2 Examples of drug concentration curve in the blood over the time: (A) high bioavailability with rapid elimination, (B) inadequate subsequent doses, and (C) doses mostly below the subtherapeutic level.

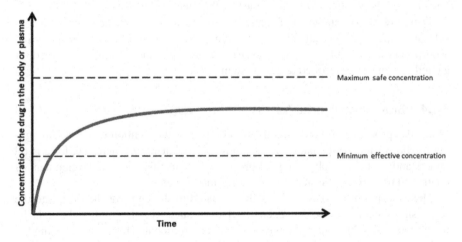

FIGURE 3.3 Example of controlled drug release curve.

by conventional forms (USP 2014). Thus, MRPFs are developed to enable better use of the drug by the body. In addition to optimizing the distribution of the API throughout the body, MRPFs avoid undesirable concentration fluctuations and allow an improvement in bioavailability.

The purpose of a DDS is to confine the API and direct it to the desired location in a protected and/or prolonged manner, releasing the API into the body. This technology has different terminologies, which will differ according to the specific product, its performance characteristics, and according to the author (Bruschi 2015). Knowing some of these terms is important for understanding these systems:

- Repeated action – the system contains more than one dose, where the first is released shortly after administration and the second or third dose is released at other time intervals;
- Controlled release – the release of the API occurs at a constant rate and provides plasma concentrations that remain invariant over the time;
- Action/sustained release – the release of the API occurs as soon as it is administered to reach a therapeutic dose and then subsequent doses are released gradually over a prolonged period;
- Delayed release – API release occurs at some point after administration;
- Prolonged release – the release of the API is maintained for a longer period after administration, thus reducing the frequency of administration and maintaining the API in plasma concentrations at a therapeutic level.

Although there are different types of DDS (Figure 3.1), the most common is the tablet dosage form, which we will treat as a traditional DDS. To better understand what DDS is, we will start with traditional DDS and end with 3D printed DDS technology. It is known that the absorption of traditional DDS largely occurs in the intestine, which is why it is important to have prior knowledge of the Biopharmaceutical Classification System (BCS) (Amidon et al. 1995). However, based on this prior knowledge it is possible to develop other orally effective DDS.

Therefore, the development of controlled release systems must be carried out considering some physiological factors of the organism that can influence the speed and absorption rate. Therefore, some biopharmaceutical parameters must be studied for a good design of a controlled release system.

3.1.4 Biopharmaceutical Aspects

Molecular processes, organs, and tissues control the distribution of drugs throughout the body and are the basis for the study of biopharmacy. Therefore, for a good understanding of how physiological processes are intrinsic to the development of controlled drug release systems, some terms must be elucidated.

The absorption of APIs in the body is related to the entry of the drug into the organism and this can be influenced by factors such as permeability through the membrane and solubility in the physiological environment. Thus, after entering the body, the drug will be distributed through the bloodstream with the aim of reaching the target tissue. This distribution can be influenced by factors such as blood perfusion in the tissue, permeability, and tissue mass. The elimination of the drug will be done by chemical transformation (metabolization) or physical removal from the body (excretion) through bile, the intestines, and/or kidneys.

The bioavailability is the amount of drug available at the site of action, thus, it describes the speed and extent that a drug is absorbed, and is a critical factor in the development of delivery systems. However, most studies do not allow the determination of the drug in the target tissue. Therefore, bioavailability studies are carried out by determining the drug concentration in the blood. This does not mean that the amount of drug in the blood and tissue are equal; however, it is considered that there is a balance of drug distribution through the bloodstream in the tissue.

The membrane permeability is defined as the speed at which a molecule moves across a membrane and is related to the resistance that a drug must cross it. Thus, the lower the resistance to membrane crossing, the greater the permeability of the drug. This permeability is determined by the solubility of the API in this membrane, transport through cellular transporters, and the thickness of the membrane.

Thus, the absorption of a drug by a biological membrane can be mediated by carriers in the membrane or by simple diffusion. The last one is determined by the transfer of a drug from a region of high concentration (e.g., gastrointestinal tract) to one of low concentration (e.g., systemic circulation). Thus, this high concentration of the drug in the gastrointestinal environment, for example, is due to the solubility of the drug in this environment.

This solubility of the drug in the physiological environment can be expressed by the partition of the drug (calculated by the partition coefficient) between two immiscible phases. Thus, a drug will move from the blood to the target tissue if it obtains a greater affinity for the components of the cell membrane.

Based on these concepts, the APIs can be classified according to their solubility and permeability through the Biopharmaceutical Classification System (BCS) proposed by Amidon and collaborators in 1995 (Figure 3.4). Class I drugs have high permeability and high solubility and are well absorbed; its absorption rate is greater than excretion. Class II drugs have high permeability but low solubility, and

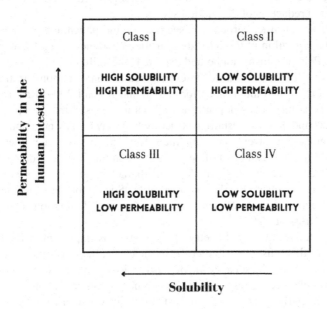

FIGURE 3.4 Classification of active pharmaceutical ingredients (APIs) according to their solubility and permeability through the biopharmaceutical classification system.

bioavailability is restricted by their solvation rate. Class III drugs have low permeability but high solubility, where the drug dissolves quickly. However, absorption is limited by the permeation rate. Class IV drugs have low permeability, low solubility, and are poorly absorbed by the intestine; therefore, they have low bioavailability with high variability (Ku 2008; Panchagnula and Thomas 2000). Thus, permeability corresponds to the ability of the API to overcome biological barriers or biological membranes and carry out the distribution, metabolism, and excretion of the drug. Solubility is important for the release and absorption of the API, as it plays a fundamental role in bioavailability.

Knowing in advance the solubility and permeability of the API is essential to begin the development of a DDS. However, they are not the only factors that can influence the absorption of API in the body, some physicochemical factors, such as the characteristics of the pharmaceutical formulation (pharmaceutical form, excipients/additives, technology involved in manufacturing the DDS) and biological characteristics such as anatomy, route of administration, and physiology also influence absorption (Hargel, Lu, and Pong 2005).

To obtain a DDS it is necessary to use an excipient/adjuvant (for solid dosage forms) or a vehicle (for semi-solid dosage forms) to stabilize the API against degradation and transport it to the desired location. They can even be used to control the speed at which the API is released and increase its bioavailability. The method used to obtain DDS influences bioavailability, such as if during the method there was agitation, a change in pH, a change in storage temperature, or in the case of tablets and capsules the use of a coating. All these factors can cause changes in EPI polymorphism and reduction of dissolution speed.

Some physicochemical properties, such as polymorphism, the particle size of an API, and the logarithm of the oil/water partition coefficient (Log P), also influence absorption. Polymorphism can be understood as the ability of a drug to exist in two or more crystalline forms with different molecular conformations, in the forms of solvates, hydrates, and amorphous forms (Lu and Rohani 2009; Raw et al. 2004). The amorphous form does not have a well-defined crystalline structure. Solvates, on the other hand, have a crystalline structure that may or may not contain stoichiometric amounts of a solvent and when the solvent involved is water, they are called hydrates. Many drugs can crystallize and transform into another polymorphic form with completely different physical–chemical characteristics, which is why analyzing the polymorphism during the development of DDS is important, since the polymorphism has been shown to influence the solubility and dissolution rate of the API (Hörter and Dressman 2001).

The particle size or granulometry of the powder is important in the dissolution of the API. In this sense, the smaller the particle size, the larger the contact surface between the API and the solvent, the better the bioavailability. Therefore, if an API is poorly soluble, decreasing its particle size may improve its solubility; however, decreasing the particle size may increase toxicity, as was seen with digoxin between 1972–1973 (Storpirtis et al. 1999). For an API to be absorbed by the body and distributed throughout body fluids, it is necessary to overcome tissue barriers that are composed of cell membranes that are lipoprotein in nature. Therefore, whether the API can diffuse through these membranes will depend on its physicochemical properties of miscibility in a predominantly oily medium. One way to know the tendency of a compound to diffuse in oil or water is to know the oil/water partition coefficient (P). The logarithm of this oil/water partition coefficient is known as Log P. Therefore, Log P = 0 indicates that the molecule has the same affinity for oil and water. Log P > 0 indicates that the molecule is lipophilic and Log P < 0 indicates that the compound is hydrophilic. Very low Log P values make permeation through cell membranes difficult. On the other hand, very high values can keep the molecules retained in the membrane, due to their high lipid solubility.

Furthermore, other biological characteristics also influence the distribution of the drug throughout the body. Some physiological factors are intrinsic to everyone, making it complex, including the circadian cycle that ends up interfering with the action of medications and with the state of the disease (Li 1987). Factors related to physiological characteristics, for example, in the case of oral DDS are, pH level, salivary enzymes, motility, gastric emptying, the presence of food and intestinal health will all influence bioavailability and dissolution speed. Topical DDS for skin is influenced by the pH level of the skin, the type of wound, the presence or lack of hair; DDS for mucosal regions (eyes, mouth, nasal mucosa, vaginal, and anal canal) suffers from the presence of fluids and secretions.

3.1.5 ADVANTAGES OF CONTROLLED DRUG DELIVERY SYSTEMS

Tablets are not the only form of drug dosage that are present in the pharmaceutical industry. Other pharmaceutical dosage forms have their space in the market. However, medicines showing traditional drug release patterns can display some disadvantages:

- Need of frequent administration;
- Very high chances of missing a dose due to forgetting;
- Difficulty monitoring daily doses;
- Difficulty in monitoring and calculating the correct dosage, especially in children and the elderly, facilitating overdose;
- Difficulty in maintaining doses within the therapeutic window;
- Difficulty in targeting an action site;
- High doses, in addition to being toxic, can cause damage to organs and cells.

Although very popular, the disadvantages need to be overcome to improve pharmacokinetics and achieve pharmacodynamics. New DDSs are being developed with the aim of guaranteeing the safety and increasing the effectiveness of APIs in drug treatment. To do this, they must have the following characteristics:

- Maintain the therapeutic level in a desired range;
- Promote bioavailability and reduce fluctuations in API concentrations in the body;

- Ensure the delivery of APIs with low or very high solubility to the desired target;
- Ensure safe dosage, ensuring that there is no low or overdose;
- Reduce daily dosages, prolonging the effect of the API within the safe therapeutic window;
- Reduce side effects and toxicity;
- Minimize or prevent local and/or systemic side effects;
- Reduce costs and ensure patient adherence to treatment;
- Reduce the accumulation of the API in the body in a possible chronic treatment;
- Enable personalized dosing for the patient.

To achieve these objectives, topical DDS that is capable of carrying APIs and guarantees their permeation and bioavailability have been developed, as we will see in the following sections.

3.2 DOSAGE FORMS FOR TOPICAL AND MUCOSAL ADMINISTRATION

Based on the biopharmaceutical factors and the definition of controlled drug release systems discussed previously, some of the main types of drug delivery systems should be exemplified. In this section, we will focus on bioadhesive delivery systems (which will be further addressed in the next chapter). Therefore, their concept is the interaction with some biological surfaces, such as the skin and mucosa.

The skin is one of the most accessible organs of the human body and can be utilized to achieve different effects, such as superficial, local, or systemic effects. When a topical DDS is applied to the skin, an interaction occurs between the formulation, the skin, and the API. This interaction and subsequent penetration of the API into the skin will follow Fickian diffusion, which occurs depending on the concentration of the active ingredient, the size of the area of contact with the skin surface, and the permeability of the skin. Skin permeability depends on some factors that must be taken into consideration when developing a topical DDS, such as the excipients used (with occlusive, moisturizing, and/or drying effects), as these, alone or in combination, modulate the release of the API (Bhowmik et al. 2012).

Even if the application is on the skin, the API can act locally, that is, in the layers of the skin (topical action) or fall into the blood system (systemic action). In transdermal pharmaceutical forms, the skin is an alternative, non-invasive route of administration, which has systemic action. For a better understanding of the pharmaceutical forms that can be applied to the skin, some terms need to be clarified and clarified, such as the difference between penetration, permeation, and absorption:

- Penetration: the API can penetrate the stratum corneum of the first layer of the skin, reaching the most superficial layers of the epidermis. Penetration can also be called skin absorption.

- Permeation: the API can act in deeper layers, reaching the dermis; however, it does not reach the blood vessels. Permeation can also be called transcutaneous absorption.
- Absorption: the API reaches the blood system in this case.

DDS for topical and mucosal applications can be in semi-solid forms (emulsions, gels, emulgels, ointments, pastes), liquid (nanostructured lipid carriers, liposomes, aerosols, eye drops), or solid (microneedles, transdermal patches, structures 3D printed).

3.2.1 SEMI-SOLID DOSAGE FORMS

3.2.1.1 Emulsions

Emulsions are pharmaceutical forms that contain water and hydrocarbons (waxes or polyols) as the base for the drugs. They are easy to obtain, and the cost depends on the hydrocarbon used. They are classified into two types: water-in-oil (W:O – system with more oil than water) or oil-in-water (O:W – system with more water than oil). Some may ask how is this possible since oil and water don't mix? Well, for this to happen it is necessary to use emulsifying agents (surfactants), which will allow the oil and water to mix, forming the emulsion. These systems can incorporate water-soluble or hydrophobic APIs and are also capable of keeping the skin hydrated and preventing water loss through the stratum corneum. They are usually white or slightly yellow. Examples of emulsions are creams and lotions.

3.2.1.2 Gels and Emulgels

Gels are obtained when the polymer (agent that gives the consistency), whether natural and/or synthetic, is incorporated into water. When swelling in water, the polymer can absorb 10 to 20% of the water and form a gel, generally translucent or slightly whitish (Hoffman 2012; Yonese 2001). The use of this type of DDS is increasing more and more, because the polymers are biodegradable, biocompatible, and safe.

When there is a combination between the emulsion and the gel, we obtain the so-called emulgel. In recent years, this system has been gaining interest in the scientific field, as polymers with these complex functions (emulsifier and thickener) allow the development of more stable emulsions, with lower surface tension, increasing the viscosity of the aqueous phase (Khullar et al. 2011; Sharma et al. 2018). Additionally, emulgel benefits from the qualities of a gel and an emulsion, making it a great DDS.

In the presence of suitable polymers, these DDS enable the application of APIs in a bioadhesive and thermoresponsive way. Basically, these terms refer to the ability of DDS to adhere to the skin or mucosa so that even with physiological movements the systems do not detach from the desired location (bioadhesive), so when applied to the mucosa this system becomes called mucoadhesive.

The term thermoresponsive is used when the DDS is applied to the desired location (skin or mucosa) and then undergoes a change in its viscosity due to an external stimulus, in this case body temperature (da Silva, Cook, and Bruschi 2020; De Souza

Ferreira et al. 2015; Jones et al. 2009). These bio/mucoadhesive and/or thermore-sponsive characteristics are leading to the emergence of new DDSs, such as nose-to-brain DDS, which aim to carry the API directly to the brain using the nasal route (Espinoza et al. 2019).

3.2.1.3   Others

Other systems such as ointments and pastes have in their composition an amount of substances insoluble (waxes, petroleum jelly, lanolin, zinc oxide) in water. They are generally used when the aim of treatment is occlusion (Bhowmik et al. 2012) and are products used in many dermatological and cosmetic skin therapies. Ointments and pastes are semi-solid formulations; however, there are differences between them. The ointment has a slightly softer consistency than paste and is made up of mono-phasic excipients with lipophilic or hydrophilic characteristics. While the paste is made up of a high percentage of insoluble solids, generally of mineral origin (zinc oxide, magnesium carbonate, calcium carbonate, titanium dioxide, among others) or vegetable origin (starches or lycopodium). These systems create a hydrophobic barrier on the skin and contribute to the matrix between the corneocytes. Its main limitations include odor, potential allergenicity, and the greasy feel associated with most occlusives. These occlusive substances are believed to diffuse into intercellular lipid domains, thus contributing to their effectiveness.

3.2.2   LIQUID DOSAGE FORMS

3.2.2.1   Lipid Nanoparticles

Liposomes have a structure and morphology in one or multiple lipid bilayers, such as cell membranes, making them an excellent option for DDSs (Figure 3.5) (Bozzuto and Molinari 2015; Zuddam et al. 2003). This lipid bilayer is located around a central aqueous compartment (core), resulting in a DDS capable of trapping lipophilic (in its

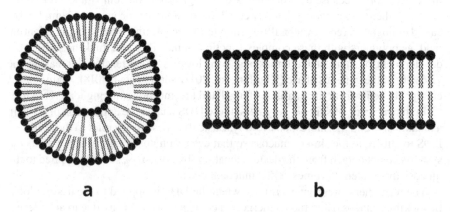

a   **b**

FIGURE 3.5   Representation of the liposome lipid bilayer (a) and the cellular lipid bilayer (b).

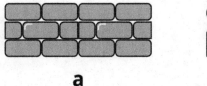 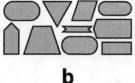

a   b

FIGURE 3.6   Representation of two types of lipid nanoparticles: (a) solid lipid nanoparticles, (b) nanostructured lipid carriers.

membrane) and hydrophilic (in its aqueous core) API. Its nano or micrometric size and morphology allow this system to be applied topically, allowing the absorption, retention, and/or permeation of the API.

There are two main types of lipid nanoparticles, solid lipid nanoparticles (SLNs) and nanostructured lipid carriers (NLCs). They came with the intention of overcoming some of the limitations of other types of colloidal carriers (emulsions, liposomes). SLNs were the first nanoparticles to be developed and present benefits in the release profile and DDS with good physical stability (Ali et al. 2016; Bozzuto and Molinari 2015).

Over time, studies began to show that these systems have some disadvantages such as low encapsulation capacity, release of drugs to the external environment, and change in viscosity during storage and transport due to their well-organized structure. To overcome these disadvantages, a new generation of lipid nanoparticles has emerged, called nanostructured lipid carriers (NLCs). To obtain NLCs, a mixture of lipids with different structures (liquid and solid lipids) are used, causing imperfections and disorganization in the structure, leaving it with a greater storage capacity for APIs (Figure 3.6) (Katouzian et al. 2017; Müller et al. 2007; Uchida et al. 2021).

3.2.2.2   Aerosols

Aerosols are DDSs capable of carrying APIs through the respiratory tract. The use of this system was intensified around the 1950s to carry antibiotics, such as penicillin (Kanig 1963; Kuhn 2002). Carrying the API through the respiratory route, mainly by nebulization, avoids systemic toxicity, and ensures that the API reaches the lungs in a concentrated form.

Patients tend to prefer the painless route of administering the medication. For this reason, pharmaceutical aerosols have been studied to meet this patient demand. However, it is not just for the respiratory route that this type of DDS is used, nowadays aerosols are being developed for the topical route (Patra, Bhattacharya, and Patnaik 2017). Although aerosol dosage forms have numerous benefits, several health and ecological concerns have also been widely reported. The aerosol spray allows the API to be applied to a wound without direct contact with a cotton swab, in other cases without the need for the use of a tongue depressor, thus minimizing waste and contamination of the formulation, covering a large area of contact, allowing better absorption of the API, and avoiding trauma to the patient (Jáuregui et al. 2009).

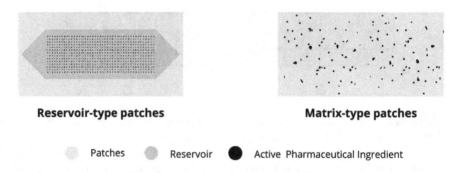

Reservoir-type patches   **Matrix-type patches**

Patches   Reservoir   Active Pharmaceutical Ingredient

FIGURE 3.7   Incorporation system of active pharmaceutical ingredient (API) in two types of patches: reservoir-type patches and in matrix-type patches.

3.2.3 Solids

For DDSs used for topical or mucosal uses microneedles, transdermal patches, and 3D printed structures are available. Patching is a DDS option. Its use is to release an API locally or systemically. The absorption of API by the skin, in this type of DDS, can be affected by the location where the patch is applied, integrity of the epidermis, molecular size of the API, pH level, blood flow, skin hydration, among others (Santos et al. 2018).

In reservoir-type patches, the API is in a solution or gel within a reservoir, and its delivery is governed by a rate-controlling membrane positioned between the patch reservoir and the skin. On the other hand, in matrix-type patches, the API is incorporated into the patches themselves (Figure 3.7) (Suedee et al. 2008).

As transdermal DDSs suffer from the barrier of the skin's stratum corneum, microneedles emerged to overcome this limitation, as they have a structure full of micro-sized needles, which, when applied to the skin, make micro-punctures in the skin in a minimally invasive way, which facilitates the penetration of the API transdermally (Vecchi et al. 2022). Microneedles can be obtained using a hydrogel base applied to a pre-molded shape or even by 3D printing using different printing methodologies (extrusion, stereolithography, filament) (Farias et al. 2018; Gittard et al. 2010; Luzuriaga et al. 2018; Shin and Hyun 2021; Vecchi et al. 2022). Microneedles can be developed in four ways (Figure 3.8):

1 Solid microneedles for skin pretreatment to increase skin permeability;
2 Microneedles coated with an API that dissolves in the skin and releases the API;
3 Polymer microneedles that encapsulate the API and completely dissolve in the skin;
4 Hollow microneedles for infusing medicine into the skin.

3D printed films come to revolutionize the area of new DDS. They can be obtained through various types of printers as seen in the previous chapter. The printed

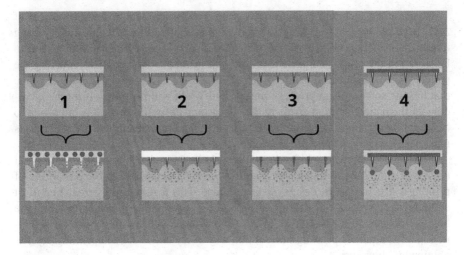

FIGURE 3.8 Types of microneedles: (1) Solid microneedles, (2) coated microneedles, (3) soluble microneedles, (4) hollow microneedles.

structures are obtained from hydrogels capable of forming pharmaceutical films. What makes the method more interesting is the ability to incorporate the API into the hydrogel and print the desired structure in a personalized way. The following sections will talk more about these 3D printed materials.

3.3 APPLICABILITY IN 3D PRINTING

The development of a DDS to carry precise amounts of an API and reduce daily dosages has attracted attention in the pharmaceutical and medical fields. The applicability of additive manufacturing (AM) has been intensely studied in the pharmaceutical and biomedical areas. Studies have demonstrated that this technology can overcome the limitations presented by traditional treatments, making it a great potential for new DDS.

However, for the 3D printing of a material to meet expectations, it is necessary, such as prior knowledge of the location where this printed material will be applied; which type of 3D printer will be the most practical and functional (see Chapter 1); what is the best polymer (natural and/or synthetic) to be used to obtain printing ink (see Chapter 5); and what is the best format, size, and dosage of API.

The use of AM as an innovative DDS presents challenges similar to traditional methods and are related to space, time, and shape. In other words, the effective and safe delivery of the API to the desired location must not only be controlled quantitatively, when applying a DDS it must be free from space restrictions and obstacles; it must be delivered in a short time and maintain the dosage in the therapeutic range; and it must be printed in ideal formats, in order to offer the best treatment and increase patient adherence.

Advances in technology, mainly in software development and improvement of AM, have allowed 3D printing to produce personalized and higher quality drug treatments. The possibility of using cloud and robotic technologies allows data to be stored in the cloud and to be retrieved and printed from anywhere, meeting the patient's needs wherever they are (Eo et al. 2018). Therefore, any pharmacy or clinic that has the software and printer connected to Wi-Fi will be able to print the medicine for the patient without errors in the dosage and desired format. It is important to highlight that to guarantee quality, effectiveness, and reproducibility the 3D printers must have excellent printing resolution.

For the development of pharmaceutical dosage forms for topical and mucosal administration, 3D printing has proven to be very effective due to the possibility of printing a structure in the desired size and shape. This feature brings greater comfort and patient compliance, as the application is easy and painless. When choosing the best 3D printer, it is essential to choose the printer with the best printing resolution and the smallest printing nozzle, this way every detail of each printing layer is obtained with precision.

The main 3D printed DDS, for the purpose of topical and mucosal applications, are pharmaceutical films and microneedle adhesives. These dosage forms can be used to carry APIs for the treatment of burns and muscle pain, to improve the healing process, to carry the API transdermally, and to deliver vaccines, among other applications (Barnum et al. 2020; Elbadawi et al. 2021; Fajardo et al. 2013; Garg et al. 2005; Gittard et al. 2010; Kim et al. 2012; Luzuriaga et al. 2018; Tsegay et al. 2022; Wang et al. 2019; Yeo et al. 2017).

For certain applications, local administration of antibiotics is more advantageous compared to systemic administration of the antibiotic, providing relatively higher therapeutic efficacy and lower systemic toxicity, which is why 3D printed DDSs prove to be effective (Palo et al. 2017). The possibility of printing microneedles with different sizes, types of entrapment, and release of APIs (Figure 3.6) makes it a good alternative for topical treatments (Luzuriaga et al. 2018). In addition to its applicability with modified release, it is easily obtained and convenient for the patient, the printed DDS has other advantages that can be seen in the next section.

3.4 ADVANTAGES OF 3D PRINTING FOR DRUG DELIVERY

The main advantages of AM for DDSs are related to the possibility of offering the patient a more individualized and personalized treatment. This personalized treatment is extremely important, considering the genetic variations of everyone in the response to treatment (Hamburg and Collins 2010).

AM allows the manufacture and development of DDSs with varied geometries and sizes, making it possible to develop DDSs with modified drug release profiles that are often difficult to achieve using conventional techniques. The drug release kinetics can be controlled by the design of the DDS., This is acheived mainly be the choice of polymers used, taking into account the polymer combinations and selecting the ideal printer, taking into account the physical and chemical characteristics of the API, that is, preventing a thermosensitive API from being printed on a 3D printer using filament (Palo et al. 2017; Uchida and Bruschi 2023).

In a 3D printed DDS, the dosage can be adjusted according to the individual needs of the patient and depending on the concentration of the dosage used, the size and format of the printed material can be changed. The ease and versatility of this new DDS technology allows for the independent tailoring and administration of multiple APIs in a 3D printed DDS, making it suitable for patient groups requiring multiple medications simultaneously (Khaled et al. 2015a, 2015b; Zhu et al. 2020). These printed DDSs can be printed with complex internal structures and compartmentalized matrix systems, which facilitate the incorporation of different APIs that can be released in a controlled manner.

Furthermore, 3D printing a new DDS depends greatly on the polymers used. One of the advantages of using the appropriate polymer is obtaining a bioadhesive system that is capable of being 3D printed and adhering to the skin or mucosa effectively, without reapplication or loss of printed material in the desired location. In the next chapter, we will understand a little more about bioadhesive systems and the possibility of them being printed by 3D technology.

REFERENCES

Ali, Z., E. B. Türeyen, Y. Karpat, and M. Çakmakci. 2016. "Fabrication of Polymer Micro Needles for Transdermal Drug Delivery System Using DLP Based Projection Stereo-Lithography." *Procedia CIRP* 42: 87–90.

Amidon, G. L., H. Lennernäs, V. P. Shah, and J. R. Crison. 1995. "A Theoretical Basis for a Biopharmaceutic Drug Classification: The Correlation of in Vitro Drug Product Dissolution and in Vivo Bioavailability." *Pharmaceutical Research* 12 (3): 413–20. Accessed October 8, 2023. https://doi.org/10.1023/A:1016212804288.

Barnum, L., M. Samandari, T. A. Schmidt, and A. Tamayol. 2020. "Microneedle Arrays for the Treatment of Chronic Wounds." *Expert Opinion on Drug Delivery* 17 (12): 1767. https://doi.org/10.1080/17425247.2020.1819787.

Bhowmik, D., H. Gopinath, B. P. Kumar, S. Duraivel, and K. P. S. Kumar. 2012. "Topical Drug Delivery system." *The Pharma Innovation* 1 (9): 12–31. Accessed October 1, 2023. https://www.researchgate.net/publication/304716203.

Bozzuto, G., and A. Molinari. 2015. "Liposomes as Nanomedical Devices." *International Journal of Nanomedicine* 10 (February): 975–99. Accessed October 3, 2023. https://doi.org/10.2147/IJN.S68861.

Bruschi, M. L. 2015. *Modification of Drug Release. Strategies to Modify the Drug Release from Pharmaceutical Systems.* Vol. 1. Elsevier. Accessed October 8, 2023. https://doi.org/10.1016/B978-0-08-100092-2.00002-3.

Elbadawi, M., D. Nikjoo, T. Gustafsson, S. Gaisford, and A. W. Basit. 2021. "Pressure-Assisted Microsyringe 3D Printing of Oral Films Based on Pullulan and Hydroxypropyl Methylcellulose." *International Journal of Pharmaceutics* 595: 120197. Accessed June 4, 2023. https://doi.org/10.1016/J.IJPHARM.2021.120197.

Eo, J., B. Cepeda, J. Kim, and N. Kim. 2018. "A New Paradigm of Pharmaceutical Drug Delivery Systems (DDS): Challenges for Space, Time, and Shapes." *Innovations in Pharmacy* 9 (3): 1. Accessed October 5, 2023. https://doi.org/10.24926/IIP.V9I3.1450.

Espinoza, L. C., M. Silva-Abreu, B. Clares, M. J. Rodríguez-Lagunas, L. Halbaut, M. A. Cañas, and A. C. Calpena. 2019. "Formulation Strategies to Improve Nose-to-Brain Delivery of Donepezil." *Pharmaceutics* 11 (2). Accessed October 3, 2023. https://doi.org/10.3390/PHARMACEUTICS11020064.

Fajardo, A. R., L. C. Lopes, A. O. Caleare, E. A. Britta, C. V. Nakamura, A. F. Rubira, and E. C. Muniz. 2013. "Silver Sulfadiazine Loaded Chitosan/Chondroitin Sulfate Films for a Potential Wound Dressing Application." *Materials Science & Engineering C, Materials for Biological Applications* 33 (2): 588–95.

Farias, C., R. Lyman, C. Hemingway, H. Chau, A. Mahacek, E. Bouzos, and M. Mobed-Miremadi. 2018. "Three-Dimensional (3D) Printed Microneedles for Microencapsulated Cell Extrusion." *Bioengineering* 5 (3): 59. https://doi.org/10.3390/BIOENGINEERING5030059.

FDA. 2015. "FOOD AND DRUG ADMINISTRATION COMPLIANCE PROGRAM GUIDANCE MANUAL PROGRAM CHAPTER 56-DRUG QUALITY ASSURANCE." 2015.

Garg, S., K. Vermani, A. Garg, R. A. Anderson, W. B. Rencher, and L. J. D. Zaneveld. 2005. "Development and Characterization of Bioadhesive Vaginal Films of Sodium Polystyrene Sulfonate (PSS), a Novel Contraceptive Antimicrobial Agent." *Pharmaceutical Research* 22 (4): 584–95.

Gittard, S. D., A. Ovsianikov, B. N. Chichkov, A. Doraiswamy, and R. J. Narayan. 2010. "Two-Photon Polymerization of Microneedles for Transdermal Drug Delivery." *Expert Opinion on Drug Delivery* 7 (4): 513–33. Accessed June 4, 2023. https://doi.org/10.1517/17425241003628171.

Hamburg, M. A., and F. S. Collins. 2010. "The Path to Personalized Medicine." *New England Journal of Medicine* 363 (4): 301–4. Accessed October 5, 2023. https://doi.org/10.1056/NEJMP1006304/SUPPL_FILE/NEJMP1006304_DISCLOSURES.PDF.

Hargel, L., A. B. C. Lu, and S. W. Pong. 2005. *Applied Biopharmaceutics & Pharmacokinetics.* 5th Ed. New York: Appleton & Lange Reviews, MacGraw-Hill.

Hoffman, A. S. 2012. "Hydrogels for Biomedical Applications." *Advanced Drug Delivery Reviews* 64 (SUPPL.): 18–23.

Hörter, D., and J. B. Dressman. 2001. "Influence of Physicochemical Properties on Dissolution of Drugs in the Gastrointestinal Tract." *Advanced Drug Delivery Reviews* 46 (1–3): 75–87. Accessed September 21, 2023. https://pubmed.ncbi.nlm.nih.gov/11259834/.

Jáuregui, K. M. G., J. C. C. Cabrera, E. P. S. Ceniceros, J. L. M. Hernández, and A. Ilyina. 2009. "A New Formulated Stable Papin-Pectin Aerosol Spray for Skin Wound Healing." *Biotechnology and Bioprocess Engineering* 14 (4): 450–56. Accessed October 3, 2023. https://doi.org/10.1007/S12257-008-0268-0/METRICS.

Jones, D. S., M. L. Bruschi, O. de Freitas, M. P. D. Gremião, E. H. G. Lara, and G. P. Andrews. 2009. "Rheological, Mechanical and Mucoadhesive Properties of Thermoresponsive, Bioadhesive Binary Mixtures Composed of Poloxamer 407 and Carbopol 974P Designed as Platforms for Implantable Drug Delivery Systems for Use in the Oral Cavity." *International Journal of Pharmaceutics* 372 (1–2): 49–58.

Kanig, J. L. 1963. "Pharmaceutical Aerosols." *Journal of Pharmaceutical Sciences* 52 (6): 513–35. Accessed October 3, 2023. https://doi.org/10.1002/JPS.2600520603.

Katouzian, I., A. Faridi Esfanjani, S. M. Jafari, and S. Akhavan. 2017. "Formulation and Application of a New Generation of Lipid Nano-Carriers for the Food Bioactive Ingredients." *Trends in Food Science & Technology* 68: 14–25. Accessed October 3, 2023. https://doi.org/10.1016/J.TIFS.2017.07.017.

Khaled, S. A., J. C. Burley, M. R. Alexander, J. Yang, and C. J. Roberts. 2015a. "3D Printing of Tablets Containing Multiple Drugs with Defined Release Profiles." *International Journal of Pharmaceutics* 494 (2): 643–50. Accessed October 5, 2023. https://doi.org /10.1016/J.IJPHARM.2015.07.067.

Khaled, S. A., J. C. Burley, M. R. Alexander, J. Yang, and C. J. Roberts. 2015b. "3D Printing of Five-in-One Dose Combination Polypill with Defined Immediate and Sustained Release Profiles." *Journal of Controlled Release* 217 (November): 308–14. https://doi .org/10.1016/J.JCONREL.2015.09.028.

Khullar, R., S. Saini, N. Seth, and A. Rana. 2011. "EMULGELS: A SURROGATE APPROACH FOR TOPICALLY USED HYDROPHOBIC DRUGS." *International Journal of Pharmacy and Biological Sciences* 1 (3): 117–28. Accessed October 1, 2023. www.ijpbs.com.

Kim, Y. C., J. H. Park, and M. R. Prausnitz. 2012. "Microneedles for Drug and Vaccine Delivery." *Advanced Drug Delivery Reviews* 64 (14): 1547–68. Accessed October 3, 2023. https://doi.org/10.1016/J.ADDR.2012.04.005.

Ku, M. S. 2008. "Use of the Biopharmaceutical Classification System in Early Drug Development." *The AAPS Journal* 10 (1): 208.

Kuhn, R. J. 2002. "Pharmaceutical Considerations in Aerosol Drug Delivery." *Pharmacotherapy: The Journal of Human Pharmacology and Drug Therapy* 22 (3P2): 80S–85S. Accessed October 3, 2023. https://doi.org/10.1592/PHCO.22.6.80S.33907.

Li, V. H. Kr. J. R. 1987. "Influence of Drug Pproperties and Routes of Drug Administration on the Design of Susteined and Controlled Release Systems." In *Controlled Drug Delivery. Fundamentals and Applications*, edited by Joseph R. Robinson and Vicent H. L. Lee, 2nd Ed. New York: Taylor & Francis Group.

Lu, J., and S. Rohani. 2009. "Polymorphism and Crystallization of Active Pharmaceutical Ingredients (APIs)." *Current Medicinal Chemistry* 16: 884–905.

Luzuriaga, M. A., D. R. Berry, J. C. Reagan, R. A. Smaldone, and J. J. Gassensmith. 2018. "Biodegradable 3D Printed Polymer Microneedles for Transdermal Drug Delivery." *Lab on a Chip* 18 (8): 1223–30. https://doi.org/10.1039/C8LC00098K.

Müller, R. H., R. D. Petersen, A. Hommoss, and J. Pardeike. 2007. "Nanostructured Lipid Carriers (NLC) in Cosmetic Dermal Products." *Advanced Drug Delivery Reviews* 59 (6): 522–30. Accessed October 3, 2023. https://doi.org/10.1016/J.ADDR.2007.04.012.

Palo, M., J. Holländer, J. Suominen, J. Yliruusi, and N. Sandler. 2017. "3D Printed Drug Delivery Devices: Perspectives and Technical Challenges." *Expert Review of Medical Devices* 14 (9): 685–96. Accessed October 5, 2023. https://www.tandfonline.com/doi/ abs/10.1080/17434440.2017.1363647.

Panchagnula, R., and N. S. Thomas. 2000. "Biopharmaceutics and Pharmacokinetics in Drug Research." *International Journal of Pharmaceutics* 201 (2): 131–50. Accessed September 21, 2023. https://pubmed.ncbi.nlm.nih.gov/10878321/.

Patra, M., S. Bhattacharya, and M. Patnaik. 2017. "Importance of Propellants and Excipients in Pharmaceutical Topical Aerosol." *Current Drug Delivery* 14 (8): 1106–13.

Raw, A. S., M. S. Furness, D. S. Gill, R. C. Adams, F. O. Holcombe, and L. X. Yu. 2004. "Regulatory Considerations of Pharmaceutical Solid Polymorphism in Abbreviated New Drug Applications (ANDAs)." *Advanced Drug Delivery Reviews* 56 (3): 397–414. Accessed September 21, 2023. https://pubmed.ncbi.nlm.nih.gov/14962589/.

Santos, L. F., I. J. Correia, A. S. Silva, and J. F. Mano. 2018. "Biomaterials for Drug Delivery Patches." *European Journal of Pharmaceutical Sciences* 118: 49–66. Accessed October 3, 2023. https://doi.org/10.1016/J.EJPS.2018.03.020.

Sharma, V., S. K. Nayak, S. R. Paul, B. Choudhary, S. S. Ray, and K. Pal. 2018. "Emulgels." In *Polymeric Gels. Characterization, Properties and Biomedical Applications*, 251–64. Woodhead Publishing. Accessed October 1, 2023. https://doi.org/10.1016/B978-0-08-102179-8.00009-0.

Shin, D., and J. Hyun. 2021. "Silk Fibroin Microneedles Fabricated by Digital Light Processing 3D Printing." *Journal of Industrial and Engineering Chemistry* 95: 126–33.

Silva, J. B. da, M. T. Cook, and M. L. Bruschi. 2020. "Thermoresponsive Systems Composed of Poloxamer 407 and HPMC or NaCMC: Mechanical, Rheological and Sol-Gel Transition Analysis." *Carbohydrate Polymers* 240: 116268.

Souza Ferreira, S. B. De, T. D. Moço, F. B. Borghi-Pangoni, M. V. Junqueira, and M. L. Bruschi. 2015. "Rheological, Mucoadhesive and Textural Properties of Thermoresponsive Polymer Blends for Biomedical Applications." *Journal of the Mechanical Behavior of Biomedical Materials* 55: 164–78.

Storpirtis, S., P. G. de Oliveira, D. Rodrigues, and D. Maranho. 1999. "Biopharmaceutical Considerations in the Manufacturing of Generic Drug Products: Aspects Related to Drug Dissolution and Absorption." *RBCF, Revista Brasileira de Ciências Farmacêuticas (Impr.)*, 1–16.

Suedee, R., C. Bodhibukkana, N. Tangthong, C. Amnuaikit, S. Kaewnopparat, and T. Srichana. 2008. "Development of a Reservoir-Type Transdermal Enantioselective-Controlled Delivery System for Racemic Propranolol Using a Molecularly Imprinted Polymer Composite Membrane." *Journal of Controlled Release* 129 (3): 170–78. Accessed October 3, 2023. https://pubmed.ncbi.nlm.nih.gov/18550193/.

Tsegay, F., M. Elsherif, and H. Butt. 2022. "Smart 3D Printed Hydrogel Skin Wound Bandages: A Review." *Polymers* 14 (5): 1012.

Uchida, Denise Tiemi, G. F. Siqueira, E. M. Dos Reis, F. L. Hegeto, A. M. Neto, A. V. Reis, M. L. Bruschi, M. V. Nova, and M. M. Júnior. 2021. "Design of Nanostructured Lipid Carriers Containing Cymbopogon Martinii (Palmarosa) Essential Oil against Aspergillus Nomius." *Molecules* 26 (16): 4825. Accessed May 12, 2022. https://doi.org/10.3390/MOLECULES26164825.

Uchida, D. T., and M. L. Bruschi. 2023. "3D Printing as a Technological Strategy for the Personalized Treatment of Wound Healing." *AAPS PharmSciTech* 24 (1): 1–25.

USP, U. S. P. 2014. "USP 37–NF 32 | USP-NF." United States Pharmacopoeia 37 and National Fomulary 32. Rockville: US Pharmacopoeial Convention. 2014. Accessed October 29, 2023. https://www.uspnf.com/official-text/proposal-statuscommentary/usp-37-nf-32.

Vecchi, C. F., R. S. dos Santos, J. B. da Silva, and M. L. Bruschi. 2022. "Design and Characterization of Polymeric Microneedles Containing Extracts of Brazilian Green Propolis." *Beilstein Journal of Nanotechnology* 13: 503–16. Accessed October 3, 2023. https://doi.org/10.3762/BJNANO.13.42.

Wang, L., Y. Luo, Z. Yang, W. Dai, X. Liu, J. Yang, B. Lu, and L. Chen. 2019. "Accelerated Refilling Speed in Rapid Stereolithography Based on Nano-Textured Functional Release Film." *Additive Manufacturing* 29: 100791. Accessed June 4, 2023. https://doi.org/10.1016/J.ADDMA.2019.100791.

Yeo, D. C., E. R. Balmayor, J. T. Schantz, and C. Xu. 2017. "Microneedle Physical Contact as a Therapeutic for Abnormal Scars." *European Journal of Medical Research* 22 (1): 1–9. https://doi.org/10.1186/S40001-017-0269-6.

Yonese, M. 2001. "Sustained Drug Delivery by Gels." In *Gels Handbook*, 3:230–40. Academic Press. Accessed September 25, 2023. https://doi.org/10.1016/B978-012394690-4/50115-8.

Zhu, X., H. Li, L. Huang, M. Zhang, W. Fan, and L. Cui. 2020. "3D Printing Promotes the Development of Drugs." *Biomedicine & Pharmacotherapy* 131: 110644. Accessed October 5, 2023. https://doi.org/10.1016/J.BIOPHA.2020.110644.

Zuddam, N. J., E. van Widen, R. de Vruech, and D. J. A. Crommelin. 2003. "Stability, Storage, and Sterilization of Lipossomes." In *Liposomes: A Practical Approach*, edited by V. P Torchilin and V Weissig, 2nd Ed. New York: Oxford University Press. Accessed October 1, 2023. https://books.google.com.br/books?hl=pt-BR&lr=&id=ClEJl4FIzrIC&oi=fnd&pg=PR13&dq=liposomes&ots=43lJRB06f2&sig=dqT8yMzC1DRxfTrT9abGvu2LQ9c#v=onepage&q=liposomes&f=false.

4 Bioadhesive Systems

4.1 INTRODUCTION

By determining the best administration routes, prolonging drug release, improving patient adherence to treatments, and strengthening the chemical and physical properties of the drug, the development of drug delivery systems (DDSs) contributes to the overall objective of optimizing drug administration (Vargason, Anselmo, and Mitragotri 2021; Ezike et al. 2023). Drug delivery technologies have advanced significantly in the last few years because of the development and improvement of novel strategies meant to improve drug delivery inside the body (Sahi et al. 2019; Vargason, Anselmo, and Mitragotri 2021). In recent years, the use of 3D printing technology to create complex medication delivery systems has advanced significantly. The creation of bioadhesive systems has also attracted interest due to its potential to extend and/or modify medication release profiles while maintaining therapeutic adherence. With an eye toward greater efficiency, these technological advancements show promise in tackling issues related to medication distribution (Basit and Trenfield 2022; Mohammed et al. 2021; Mohapatra et al. 2022).

The term bioadhesion describes the innate ability of two substrates, one of which is biologically derived, to stick to one another. More specifically, this interaction is called mucoadhesion when it comes to a biological substrate such as the mucous membrane (Shaikh et al. 2011; Woodley 2012; Palacio and Bhushan 2012). In many biomedical applications bioadhesion is essential. This is especially true for drug delivery systems and medical devices, where adhesion to biological surfaces extends local drug release and improves therapeutic efficacy. Gaining an understanding of and using the idea of bioadhesion has great potential for improving patient outcomes from a variety of medical procedures and expanding tailored drug delivery systems (Dey, Bhattacharya, and Neogi 2021; Woodley 2012; Porwal and Pathak 2023; Shaikh et al. 2011).

With the addition of bioadhesive polymers (natural or synthetic) this bioadhesion process may be improved or integrated into a delivery system. These polymers have special qualities that allow them to stick to biological surfaces, allowing the delivery system to stay at the intended site of action for a longer period of time (K. Kumar et al. 2014; Ugoeze 2020; L. Kumar et al. 2017). Bioadhesion is mediated by a variety of complex mechanisms, including particular receptor–ligand binding, hydrogen bonding, and electrostatic interactions. We will go into great detail about these mechanisms in this chapter, exposing their complexities and clarifying how they help promote bioadhesion in drug delivery systems (Heikal, Hammady, and Gad 2016; Shaikh et al. 2011; K.Kumar et al. 2014).

In pharmaceutical and biomedical research, the combination of bioadhesive systems and 3D printing technology offers a wide range of options to improve patient

 DOI: 10.1201/9781003442363-4

outcomes and therapeutic efficacy. Through the utilization of 3D printing's accuracy and adaptability, bioadhesive polymer may be easily incorporated into complex 3D objects with customized geometries. This integration makes it easier to create advanced drug delivery systems that can adhere to biological surfaces for prolonged periods of time, improving therapeutic benefits and drug localization (de Oliveira et al. 2023; Wu et al. 2024; K. Kumar et al. 2014).

Moreover, patient-specific dose forms can be created using 3D printing, providing individual therapies that address each patient's specific physiological variances and therapeutic demands. The optimization of formulation characteristics, such as polymer composition and spatial distribution, is another way that 3D printing's versatility can be applied. Furthermore, the novel technologies are accelerated by the scalability and quick prototyping capabilities of 3D printing, which provide accelerated development routes for bioadhesive formulations (de Oliveira et al. 2023; Chan et al. 2024; Wu et al. 2024). Thus, as this chapter will demonstrate, the combination of bioadhesive systems with 3D printing holds great potential for transforming drug delivery methods, enhancing precision medicine, and developing customized therapeutic treatments.

4.2 ADMINISTRATION ROUTES OF BIOADHESIVE SYSTEMS

Consequently, because bioadhesion has been defined as a system's capacity to adhere in a biological substrate, there are multiple routes to administer bioadhesive drug delivery systems (Figure 4.1) (Heikal, Hammady, and Gad 2016; Shaikh et al. 2011). Topical, transdermal , and mucosal delivery are particularly important routes of administration.

Therefore, more investigation and elucidation of the skin's physiology, which involves topical and transdermal delivery as well as mucus physiology, are necessary. Improved knowledge of these complex mechanisms has great potential to further drug delivery approaches, improving treatment results and patient care.

4.2.1 TOPICAL AND TRANSDERMAL ADMINISTRATION

For many years, the skin has been utilized to administer drugs for local (topical) treatment. More recently, studies have been conducted on transdermal drug delivery systems. Because it allows for specific therapy and eliminates some of the disadvantages associated with other routes of drug administration, using the skin as a drug delivery route is attracting a lot of interest in both clinical and research contexts (Ramadon et al. 2022; Jeong et al. 2021). Furthermore, new developments in formulation technology have increased the range of options for using the skin as a delivery system for drugs, enabling regulated release and improving therapeutic results.

4.2.1.1 Physiology of Skin

The skin functions as a complex barrier, producing melanin to protect the organism from UV radiation and from pathogenic risks. It has two main structural layers: the dermis and the epidermis. Keratinocytes, melanocytes, Langerhans cells, and

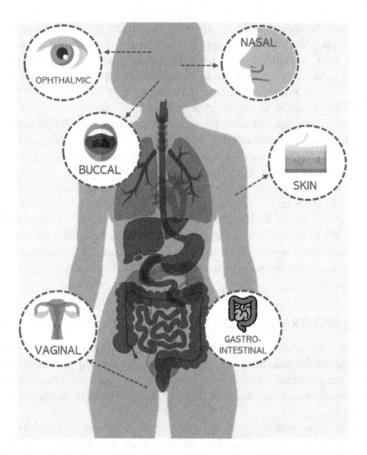

FIGURE 4.1   Main administration routes of bioadhesive systems.

Merkel cells are found in the epidermis, which is formed by epithelial tissue. The dermis, which is found below the epidermis, is rich in the extracellular matrix and is composed of collagen, elastin, proteoglycans, and fibronectin (Ramadon et al. 2022; Jeong et al. 2021).

The skin is vulnerable to damage due to its exposure to a variety of environmental variables, including mutagenic and carcinogenic effects, which grow worse from repeated exposure (Charitakis et al. 2022).

The epidermis serves multiple protective functions, including physical, chemical, biochemical, and immunological defense mechanisms. These strategies involve hydrolytic enzymes, lipids, antimicrobial peptides, and structures such as the stratum corneum and intercellular proteins. Langerhans cells are immunocompetent components that are important in immunology (Lee, Jeong, and Ahn 2006).

The skin's color, texture, and water content are also influenced by the epidermis. It is composed of four histological layers that are distinguished by the appearance and maturation of keratinocytes. The protective stratum corneum is created by keratinization and eventual apoptosis of keratinocytes that migrate from the basal layer to the superficial layers (Martini et al. 2018).

Melanocytes, which constitute approximately 8% of epidermal cells, create the pigment melanin, which is essential for both UV protection and skin color. The dermis and epidermis are linked by the dermo-epidermal junction, which is composed of layers such as the lamina lucida and lamina densa, where the neurovascular supply to the epidermis (Lee, Jeong, and Ahn 2006).

The hypodermis, located below the dermis, consists of flexible connective and adipose tissues, and works as an insulation layer and energy storage. The structure and function of the skin changes with age, resulting in a range of illnesses and consequences related to dermatology, including a higher risk of skin cancer and other diseases (Lee, Jeong, and Ahn 2006).

Topical drug administration, besides being a non-invasive route, can be advantageous when the goal is to avoid first-pass metabolism. Therefore, the development of topical delivery systems aims to treat a local or systemic disorder when the formulation has the capability of transdermal release.

4.2.2 ADMINISTRATION BY MUCOSA

The process of bioadhesion is called mucoadhesion when the biological surface involved is a mucosa. The mouth, nasal, ocular, rectal, and vaginal areas of the organism are covered in mucus. As a result, there are multiple routes to administer mucoadhesive systems.

4.2.2.1 Physiology of Mucus

Mucus performs essential functions for the organism. It constitutes of a secretion produced by specialized goblet cells that coat organs exposed to external environments. Mucus serves an essential function in preserving homeostasis and defending the body against external risks by acting as a barrier from infections and dangerous substances, allowing the flow of elements, such as nutrients, and preserving the hydration of the epithelial cell layer. Its composition is predominantly water, with mucin glycoproteins also forming a significant amount in addition to proteins, lipids, and mucopolysaccharides, although in smaller quantities (Herath et al. 2020; Johansson et al. 2011).

Furthermore, mucus is essential for the passage of materials through the nasal cavity, gastrointestinal tract, and vagina, among other anatomical places. Mucus's characteristics are influenced by physiological stimuli in different sites, requiring modifications to its composition and structure. For instance, compared to other sites, the lower airway mucus receives comparatively low mechanical forces, which causes variations in the amount of mucus produced and its rheological characteristics (Abrami et al. 2024; Boegh and Nielsen 2015).

Moreover, the specific requirements of different tissues and organs influence the anatomical distribution of mucus. Because they are constantly exposed to outside stimuli, some areas of the body, such as the respiratory and gastrointestinal tracts, produce more mucus than others. These differences are indicative of the functions that mucus plays in each anatomical site, roles that are adapted to satisfy specific physiological requirements.

The mucus barrier on epithelial surfaces functions as a crucial aspect of the innate immune system under normal physiological settings, providing a strong barrier against the penetration and absorption of foreign substances. In addition to mucins, mucus also includes lysozyme, lactoferrin, secretory IgA, lipids, polysaccharides, and different ionic species. These elements promote mucus's bacteriostatic properties and enhance its protective effects. In order to preserve tissue integrity and inhibit dangerous substances from penetrating the organism, this barrier function is essential (Sheng and Hasnain 2022; Di Sabatino et al. 2023).

Mucin molecules are kept in goblet and submucosal cells, where compact packing is made possible by calcium ions shielding the molecules. The release of calcium into the luminal area reveals these negative charges, which causes expansion and the creation of a viscoelastic gel. Mucin chains interconnect, interpenetrate, and create an organized network when there is water, which defines the mechanical characteristics of mucus (Curnutt et al. 2020).

From an engineering perspective, mucus is a great water-based lubricant that is widely found in nature. Because of its characteristics, a variety of animals use mucus to survive in challenging environments. For example, snails can cross sharp surfaces without getting cut, while giraffes can remove leaves from prickly trees. Mucus's amazing versatility and functionality in biological systems is emphasized by this natural lubricant, which has resulted in advances in biomimetic materials and drug delivery systems (Deng et al. 2023).

In conclusion, mucus is used as a flexible and dynamic defensive system, keeping the body hydrated, preventing bacterial infections, regulating immunological responses, and protecting the body from external dangers. Understanding the complicated interactions among mucus production, structure, and function at various anatomical sites is crucial to understanding the variety of functions that mucus has in health and disease.

4.2.2.2 Mucus Production

The process of producing mucus involves several cell types that are dispersed throughout the mucosal surfaces of the body. The principal mucus-producing cells in the eyes, nasal cavity, bronchial tract, and gastrointestinal system are intraepithelial mucus cells, specifically goblet cells. Mucus is secreted by these cells to form barriers that shield the body from irritants and infections outside. In addition, certain cell types including mucus cells in the endocervix and foveolar cells in the stomach, also aid in the formation of mucus in particular tissues (Davis and Wypych 2021).

The production of the mucus layer that forms the tear film in the eye is mostly dependent on the intraepithelial goblet cells found in the bulbar conjunctiva. This tear film, which keeps the ocular surface properly lubricated and hydrated, is composed of a mix of mucus, aqueous secretions from the lacrimal glands, and oily secretions from the meibomian glands. Goblet cells are crucial for maintaining eye health since they have the potential to penetrate the cornea in specific situations (Dartt 1992).

Mucus in the respiratory system is produced by submucosal glands in the trachea and bronchi as well as goblet cells. Goblet cells can be found all across the respiratory system, although bigger airways are home to submucosal glands. In order to capture and eliminate foreign objects, these glands release mucus, which supports respiratory defense systems (Davis and Wypych 2021; Williams et al. 2006).

In the oral cavity, the thickness of the mucus layer is increased by saliva produced by extra mucosal glands, especially the sublingual and submaxillary glands. The oral mucosa does not include goblet cells, in contrast to other areas. Similar to this, the gastrointestinal system produces mucus through the actions of intraepithelial mucus-producing cells in the stomach and intestinal mucosa, as well as submucosal glands in the esophagus and duodenum (Davis and Wypych 2021).

Distinct anatomical regions have diverse mucus layer architectures, which reflect the necessities of each tissue. As a protective barrier, mucus, for instance, forms a single layer over the epithelial glycocalyx in the airways and on the surfaces of the eyes. Whereas mucus in the stomach and colon is composed of two layers, one adherent and impermeable to bacteria, and the other non-adherent and luminal, which is created by enzymatic processing of mucins (H. Li et al. 2015).

Acetylcholine, neuropeptides such as neurotensin and vasoactive intestinal peptide, and cytokines are among the signaling molecules that regulate mucus secretion in the gastrointestinal and respiratory tracts. Gastrin, histamine, and prostaglandins all contribute to the stimulation of mucus release, reflecting the intricate regulatory processes. While stimulated secretion requires exocytosis, which causes mucus to expand to release, basal secretion depends on the cytoskeletal mobility of secretory granules (Schubert 1979).

Overall, to preserve mucosal integrity and defend against outside dangers, mucus formation and secretion are strictly regulated processes. The complex defensive mechanisms of the body's mucosal surfaces can be better understood by taking into account the cellular and molecular processes that constitute the generation of mucus in various tissues (Song et al. 2023).

4.2.2.3   Composition, Thickness, and Turnover of Mucus

The basic composition of mucus is basically the same despite various origins and structural differences in mucus layers across tissues. Mucus is composed of a mixture of mucins, non-mucin proteins, salts, lipids, and cells. It is approximately 97% water and 3% compounds. Mucins, an example of large glycoprotein, constitute about 30% of these compounds overall (Bansil and Turner 2018; Abrami et al. 2024).

Divided into two groups, mucins are classified as membrane-associated mucins and secreted mucins. While secreted mucins greatly increase mucus's viscosity and affect its rheological characteristics, membrane-bound mucins are involved in cell adhesion, pathogen attachment, and signal transmission (Bansil and Turner 2018).

Overall, the distinct characteristics of mucus, such as its viscosity, adhesion, and barrier roles, are a result of the complex structure and content of mucins. Comprehending the molecular properties of mucins offers an important understanding of the physiological functions of mucus in diverse biological processes and disease conditions (Bansil and Turner 2018; Abrami et al. 2024; Song et al. 2023).

While there are some similarities in the rheological characteristics of mucus at different anatomical sites, mucus layer thicknesses differ significantly. For example, nasal mucus typically has a relatively thin covering, measuring between 5.5 and 15 µm, but the mucin layer on the conjunctiva of the eye measures between 0.2 and 1 µm. Between 7 to 70 µm is the range of thickness in the bigger airways. It's interesting to note that, depending on variables such as saliva volume and mouth surface area, the mucus layer in the oral cavity can vary from 70 to 100 µm (Klitgaard et al. 2024).

In the gastrointestinal tract, mucus layers are noticeably thicker, with colon mucus layers reaching up to 1 mm in thickness and cervicovaginal mucus layers measuring 200 µm. These variations in mucus thickness are indicative of the various physiological requirements and functions that are present in various anatomical sites (Macierzanka, Mackie, and Krupa 2019; Herath et al. 2020; Paone and Cani 2020).

Mucus clearance also demonstrates a significant variance. For example, tear flow is quick, clearing the eyes in a couple of seconds, but the mucous layer in the eyes takes 15 to 20 hours to regenerate. About every 20 minutes, nasal mucus turnover occurs, while mucus in the upper airways is estimated to be eliminated at a rate of 1 mm per minute (Hill et al. 2014; Knowles and Boucher 2002).

While gastrointestinal mucus regenerates completely every 20 hours, cervical mucus turnover occurs over a period of hours. Particles are eliminated within minutes to hours, depending on their anatomical site, based on the diffusion of particles and the rheological characteristics of the mucus. These differences in mucus clearance rates illustrate how dynamic mucus physiology is and how important it is to maintain homeostasis and prevent foreign invaders (Hill et al. 2014; Knowles and Boucher 2002).

4.2.3 Buccal Drug Delivery

Among the many benefits the buccal cavity offers for drug administration applications are its excellent accessibility and low enzymatic activity. Furthermore, buccal drug delivery can be quickly discontinued in cases of toxicity by removing the dosage form, resulting in a safe and simple way of medication administration. Recent studies have focused on the controlled delivery of macromolecular therapeutic agents, such as peptides, proteins, and polysaccharides, while initial generation mucoadhesives, while mucoadhesive polymers such as sodium carboxymethylcellulose, hydroxypropylcellulose, and polycarbophil have been thoroughly studied, especially for the treatment of periodontal disease (Sudhakar, Kuotsu, and Bandyopadhyay 2006).

Although gels and ointments are the most convenient for patients, tablets, patches, and films have also been tested. High patient compliance, minimal irritability, and notable ease of administration are frequently linked to drug delivery to cutaneously accessible areas, such as the buccal cavity. Other lesser-known benefits include a faster effect start time due to the highly vascularized buccal mucosa and the avoidance of hepatic first-pass metabolism (Sudhakar, Kuotsu, and Bandyopadhyay 2006).

Orabase®, a first-generation mucoadhesive material, has long been used as a barrier against mouth ulcers. Recent formulation advances have resulted in a combined corticosteroid (triamcinolone acetonide) with Orabase® product, which gives local treatment of mouth ulcers through a dual mechanism: a barrier function and an anti-inflammatory function (due to triamcinolone acetonide) (Julião et al. 2022).

Although semisolid systems are convenient and comfortable, tablets and patches often give greater active ingredient stability (typically solid-state), improved residence time, and, therefore, longer periods of therapeutic drug levels at site of action.

Multilayer systems with an adhesive layer and additional drug-functional layers have been a common feature of tablet and patch platforms. Other common engineering approaches have included matrix devices. A layer impermeable to drugs is frequently used in such devices to promote unidirectional drug delivery, hence avoiding salivary gland clearance mechanisms (Jackson and Miller 2008).

Pressing the dose form under the upper lip is a frequent method of preventing tablet clearance from the buccal cavity. This is how Buccastem®, an adhesive antiemetic pill with prochlorperazine maleate, is given. Although bioadhesive tablets have many benefits, some patients may find using these drug delivery platforms uncomfortable due to the oscillatory action of talking and mastication. This discomfort is a major reason why semisolid and flexible patch-based systems predominate buccal medication administration (Chinna Reddy, Chaitanya, and Madhusudan Rao 2011).

The oral route is the most patient-compliant way for delivering diverse therapeutic substances since it eliminates discomfort, pain, and the risk of infection. However, the efficacy of the oral route has been restricted by some related problems, such as acidic destruction of bioactive compounds in the stomach, low macromolecular permeability through intestinal epithelium, and degradation through proteolytic enzymes (Suharyani et al. 2021; Mohammadzadeh and Javadzadeh 2018; Lou et al. 2023; Homayun, Lin, and Choi 2019).

Medication administered orally might be administered sublingually or buccally. The buccal mucosa has decreased permeability, resulting in less absorption and reduced medication bioavailability, while the sublingual mucosa is very permeable, absorbing medicines quickly and increases their bioavailability. However, sublingual mucosa has been found to be unsatisfactory for bioadhesive system delivery due to its dispersion caused by regular cleaning through produced saliva. So, as a result, the buccal mucosa is preferred over sublingual mucosa for delivering bioadhesives (Chinna Reddy, Chaitanya, and Madhusudan Rao 2011; Gilhotra et al. 2014).

4.2.4 Ophthalmic Drug Delivery

Therapeutic agents can be delivered to the eye using a variety of dose forms, such as liquid drops, gels, ointments, and solid ocular inserts, both degradable and non-degradable. Another intriguing delivery platform is in situ gelling polymers, which change phase after application. These systems are in liquid condition before application, making them simple to administrate, and after application they convert into very viscous rheologically structured networks. Temperature, pH levels, and the presence of specific ions (calcium ions) in the ocular fluid are all examples of transitory stimuli (S. Li, Chen, and Fu 2023; Nhàn, Maidana, and Yamada 2023).

The non-specificity of first-generation platforms, however, is an important consideration when using mucoadhesive polymers in the eye. While mucoadhesive polymers are predicted to adhere only to conjunctival mucus in vivo, diffusion may cause semisolid deposition within the corneal region, potentially affecting visual acuity. Certain polymers have also demonstrated limited absorption in vivo due to their high swelling capacity in the eye's neutral pH environment (Račić and Krajišnik 2023; Burhan et al. 2021).

Ophthalmic solutions are the most commonly used dose type for ocular applications. They often have low bioavailability and therapeutic response due to rapid precorneal clearance of the active drug caused by high tear fluid turnover. This needs high frequency dosing, raising concerns regarding patient compliance. On the other hand, drug-loaded ocular inserts may provide more control over drug release rate and longer residence durations, patients may find them uncomfortable due to their stiffness, although may reduce user adoption and compliance (Le Bourlais et al. 1998; Castro-Balado et al. 2020).

Topical medicine administration to the eyes is generally accepted, and many ocular illnesses are treated with various topical treatments. However, physiological activity such as reflex lacrimation, blinking, and fast drainage contribute to low medication absorption in the eye. To improve ocular bioavailability, the medicines' duration in the ocular cavity should be enhanced. Semisolid formulations, such as ointments or gels, can interact with the eyes over time, although they may induce impaired vision, sticky sensations, and ocular pain (Ahmed, Amin, and Sayed 2023; Koutsoviti et al. 2021).

The concept of bioadhesion in ophthalmic dosage forms is relatively recent. Researchers investigated various bioadhesive formulations for ocular medication delivery, including bioadhesive mini-tablets and nanoparticles. These formulations have demonstrated good results in terms of mucoadhesive strength and drug release duration, suggesting potential benefits for enhancing ocular medication delivery (Baranowski et al. 2014).

4.2.5 VAGINAL DRUG DELIVERY SYSTEMS

Vaginal drug delivery stands out as a viable route for pharmaceutical administration, with numerous advantages over other methods such as parenteral delivery. These advantages include avoiding hepatic first-pass metabolism, which leads to increased drug bioavailability, as well as a significant reduction in the frequency and severity of gastrointestinal adverse effects often associated with oral delivery. Furthermore, this method reduces hepatic side effects and helps avoid discomfort, tissue damage, and infection risks associated with invasive parenteral injections (Acartürk 2009).

The vaginal site, with its large surface area, abundant blood supply, and high permeability, is an appealing location for systemic medication delivery. However, issues with inadequate retention due to the vaginal tract's self-cleaning action continue to be a concern. Despite this, medications delivered vaginally have a longer residence duration within the vaginal cavity than other absorption sites such as the rectum or intestinal mucosa (Acartürk 2009).

A variety of factors influence the efficacy and performance of vaginal dose forms. These factors include sensitivity and personal cleanliness standards and local discomfort. Furthermore, variations in the thickness of the vaginal epithelium during the menstrual cycle and postmenopausal period can affect drug absorption rates and extents (Smoleński et al. 2021; Pandey et al. 2021).

Various bioadhesive polymers, including polycarbophil, hydroxypropylcellulose, and polyacrylic acid have been studied for their usefulness in vaginal formulations in order to improve medication retention and targeted therapeutic benefits (Leyva-Gómez et al. 2018).

Mucoadhesive platforms are important in vaginal medication delivery because they include patient comfort and acceptance in addition to therapeutic efficacy, maintaining stability and uniform drug release profiles, especially in the face of physiological variability such as menstrual cycle–related changes in vaginal fluid composition. This way, the vaginal system delivery has great promise for both local and systemic applications (Osmałek et al. 2021; Acartürk 2009; Andrade, Parente, and Ares 2014).

4.2.6 NASAL DELIVERY SYSTEMS

Because of its histological advantages, the nasal mucosa is an appealing target for systemic medication administration. The nasal mucosa has a surface area of around 150 cm² and is extensively vascularized, making it an excellent absorptive interface for drugs. Its relatively porous epithelium, with only two cell layers separating the nasal lumen from the underlying vasculature, highlights its suitability for drug delivery applications. However, increased permeability makes nasal mucosa cells vulnerable to potential side effects from intranasal drugs and excipients (Bitter, Suter-Zimmermann, and Surber 2011; Fortuna, Schindowski, and Sonvico 2022).

Intranasal medication administration has a substantial advantage over first-pass metabolism because blood from the nasal cavity drains directly into systemic circulation. This promotes rapid systemic absorption of medicines, making it a promising route for therapeutic delivery. Nasal medication administration has been achieved using a variety of formulations, including solutions, powders, gels, and microparticles. This strategy offers patients a convenient and easy way to self-medicate (Keller, Merkel, and Popp 2022; Bitter, Suter-Zimmermann, and Surber 2011).

Notably, because of the nasal epithelium's high permeability and minimal enzymatic activity, nasal medication delivery has showed promise in treating disorders such as acute nausea and vomiting, as well as increasing protein and peptide absorption. Controlled-release formulations can be produced using nasal mucoadhesive polymers to extend medication release and improve therapeutic efficacy (Chaturvedi, Kumar, and Pathak 2011; Boddupalli et al. 2010; Anand, Feridooni, and Agu 2012).

Despite these benefits, difficulties such as fast clearance from the nasal cavity restrict the duration and efficacy of medication release. Researchers are investigating several polymeric components, such as hydroxypropylcellulose, chitosan, and carbomer as mucoadhesive agents to overcome these obstacles and enable regulated medication administration to nasal locations. Furthermore, combination systems that incorporate various polymers show promise for improving mucoadhesion and extending drug release kinetics (Anand, Feridooni, and Agu 2012; Chaturvedi, Kumar, and Pathak 2011; Boddupalli et al. 2010; Chonkar, Nayak, and Udupa 2015).

4.2.7 Gastrointestinal Drug Delivery Systems

The oral route stands out as the major route of delivering diverse medicinal substances, giving good patient compliance to the therapy. In contrast to parenteral approaches, oral administration does not require specialist professional, allowing patients to simply self-administer drugs. However, this route frequently faces obstacles such as low bioavailability and quick first-pass metabolism, especially with specific medicines (Homayun, Lin, and Choi 2019).

To address these problems, researchers created novel gastro-muco formulations aimed at optimizing drug release kinetics and pharmacokinetics. Umamaheshwari and colleagues, for example, investigated the use of mucoadhesive gliadin nanoparticles loaded with amoxicillin to eradicate *Helicobacter pylori*. These nanoparticles have a longer gastrointestinal (GIT) residence time due to improved mucoadhesion, leading to more efficient bacterial eradication than free medication formulations (Umamaheshwari, Ramteke, and Jain 2004).

Despite these developments, difficulties remain, such as the irregular gastrointestinal transit seen with some formulations. Peristalsis, fast mucus turnover, and encapsulation of delivery vehicles within a mucus shell all have a substantial impact on the success of mucoadhesive drug delivery platforms. However, continuing research is investigating new strategies and formulations to overcome these difficulties and realize the full potential of oral drug delivery systems (Boddupalli et al. 2010; Carvalho et al. 2010; Shaikh et al. 2011).

4.3 THEORIES OF BIOADHESION

For many years, researchers have been interested by the interaction of bioadhesion, in which delivery systems adhere to biological surfaces as skin and mucous membranes. As will be discussed in this chapter, investigating this phenomenon has resulted in the development of several theories, each focusing on a different aspect. It's essential to remain aware that the manifestation of bioadhesion might differ greatly depending on a number of variables, including the polymer's composition, administration technique, and delivery system. Because of its complexity, several bioadhesion mechanisms can work independently at times and in collaboration with other mechanisms at other times, which improves our comprehension of this phenomenon (Carvalho et al. 2010; Woodley 2012).

4.3.1 The Electrostatic Theory

According to this principle, there is a complicated interplay of electronic dynamics since the target biological tissue and the bioadhesive system carry opposing electrical charges. When they come into contact an intriguing electron exchange occurs, which results in the creation of an electrical double layer at the interface. In this electrostatic environment, the attractive forces acting on the double layer are crucial in defining the resulting bioadhesive force (Yu et al. 2022; Shaikh et al. 2011; Carvalho et al. 2010).

The electrostatic theory of bioadhesion is based on the idea that differences in the electrical configurations of the bioadhesive systems and the biological tissue facilitate the transmissions of electrons between them. The process of bioadhesion is controlled by this electron exchange. This electron transfer results in the formation of a double layer of electric charges at the interface between the biological surface and the bioadhesive system. Strong attraction forces are created in the double-layered area by this exciting event, strengthening the adhesive bond between the materials (Shaikh et al. 2011; Carvalho et al. 2010; L. Kumar et al. 2017).

Essentially, the electrostatic theory outlines a fundamental comprehension of the bioadhesive mechanism, clarifying the chemical exchanges which occur effect at the bioadhesive system and biological interface.

4.3.2 The Wettability Theory

There are several important ideas in the theory of how bioadhesive drug delivery systems interact with biological substrates, especially when it comes to spreadability and wettability. Spreadability, or a substance's capacity to disperse across a surface, is essential to bioadhesion, particularly in systems with low mucoadhesive or viscosity levels (Boddupalli et al. 2010; Carvalho et al. 2010).

In this context, the wettability theory suggests that bioadhesive systems first penetrate the substrate's irregular surface, after which, with an adhesive system, they have a tendency to diffuse across the surface, this mechanism is especially relevant to bioadhesive systems..

Additionally, the chemical composition of bioadhesive polymers affects their affinity for biological surfaces; polymers with functional groups that are similar to those in the biological layer have higher miscibility and are consequently more spreadable. This emphasizes how crucial molecular compatibility is for promoting successful bioadhesion (K. Kumar et al. 2014).

In practical terms, contact angle strategies can be used to measure a level of affinity between a bioadhesive system and a biological substrate, where smaller contact angles indicate stronger affinity. The liquid quickly distributes and hydrates the solid surface when the contact angle is zero, indicating the most effective potential association between the bioadhesive system and the biological substrate (Carvalho et al. 2010).

In general, the theory of spreadability and wettability offer significant understanding of the mechanics behind bioadhesion, influencing the development and optimization of bioadhesive drug delivery systems for increased therapeutic effectiveness.

4.3.3 The Diffusion Interpenetration Theory

According to this theory, bioadhesion results from the diffusion of bioadhesive polymer chains, which are mostly complex glycoproteins, over time into the complex network of mucus. Diffusion coefficients of the substrate and the interacting polymer influence the penetration process into the substrate (Boddupalli et al. 2010; Carvalho et al. 2010).

The cross-linking density, molecular weight, chain mobility/flexibility, and temperature are some of the variables that affect the polymer's effective penetration into the biological surface. All these factors work together to dictate how far the polymeric chains can penetrate and form sticky connections inside the biological layer (Hoti et al. 2021).

Furthermore, the theory explains that the establishing of semipermanent adhesive bonds over time depends significantly on the degree of interpenetration of mucoadhesive polymeric chains and mucin chains. According to empirical estimations, effective bioadhesive bonding usually requires an interpenetration depth of 0.2 to 0.5 µm. The diffusion coefficient and contact time are important variables in this process (Carvalho et al. 2010; Shaikh et al. 2011; Peppas, Thomas, and McGinity 2011).

Temperature dynamics are also important since higher temperatures are capable of making polymeric dispersion more fluid which makes it easier for mucin chains to interpenetrate. However, temperature increases can also damage the polymeric system's cohesion, which could reduce their adhesive properties (Carvalho et al. 2010; Boddupalli et al. 2010; Bayer 2022).

Additionally, the theory acknowledges the role that polymer chain length plays in the processes of diffusion and interpenetration. Longer polymeric chains can diffuse and interpenetrate across a larger mucosal surface area, but molecular tangling and optimal interpenetration are only achieved at critical chain lengths of at least 100,000 Da.

This comprehensive strategy essentially emphasizes the complex interactions between diffusion-based mechanisms, interpenetration depth, and environmental factors that control bioadhesive interactions. It is vital to comprehend and enhance these factors to improve the effectiveness and efficiency of bioadhesive drug delivery systems.

4.3.4 Adsorption Theory

This hypothesis explores the complex mechanics of bioadhesion and connects it to interactions between the polymer and the biological substrate on the surface. Primary and secondary bonding are the two basic groups into which these interactions fall (Peppas, Thomas, and McGinity 2011; Uma 2023; Heikal, Hammady, and Gad 2016).

Primary bonds, which include ionic, covalent, and metallic bonds, provide permanent links between the substrate and the polymer. Although they provide stability, their permanence, which may restrict flexibility and reversibility, in adhesion,makes them frequently seen as undesirable (Heikal, Hammady, and Gad 2016; Peppas, Thomas, and McGinity 2011).

On the other hand, secondary bonds are semipermanent in nature and result from hydrogen bonds, van der Waals forces, and hydrophobic interactions. Although less strong on their own, these connections work together to promote adhesion by establishing a balance between flexibility and strength. Secondary bonds are especially common in the setting of mucoadhesion (Uma 2023; Heikal, Hammady, and Gad 2016).

Therefore, the complex interaction of primary and secondary surface contacts results in adhesion. Secondary contacts facilitate reversible adhesion by offering flexibility and adaptability in contrast to primary interactions, which provide stability. Effective adhesion is made possible by this combination of bonding processes, which protects the integrity of the substrate and the polymer (Peppas, Thomas, and McGinity 2011; Heikal, Hammady, and Gad 2016).

Secondary interactions are also more easily reversible because it takes less energy to break them. On the other hand, as seen in bioadhesion process, their combined abundance can result in strong, semipermanent adhesion (Peppas, Thomas, and McGinity 2011; Heikal, Hammady, and Gad 2016).

In summary, understanding how primary and secondary bonding mechanisms interact offers important insights into the development and enhancement of bioadhesive systems, permitting the use of these materials in biomedical and drug delivery applications.

4.3.5 MECHANICAL THEORY

According to the mechanical theory of adhesion, a bioadhesive liquid fills in the gaps formed by imperfections on an abrasive surface. This hypothesis states that surface roughness is essential for increasing the interfacial area that is available for interactions. By facilitating the dissipation of energy, this increase in interfacial area promotes the formation of adhesion bonds (Carvalho et al. 2010).

Essentially, the mechanical theory emphasizes the physical aspect of adhesion, which in turn emphasizes the role that surface characteristics, such as roughness, have in promoting successful adherence. Rougher surfaces provide more surface area for molecular interactions, which enhances the adhesion connections. The bioadhesive liquid increases contact with the substrate by filling in surface imperfections, which strengthens and stabilizes the adhesion bond overall (Carvalho et al. 2010; Packham 2011).

In general, the mechanical theory of adhesion provides a basis for improving adhesion properties and performance through approaches to surface modification and the selection of suitable adhesive materials. Therefore, an understanding of these principles is crucial for the design and optimization of bioadhesive systems.

4.4 BIOADHESIVE POLYMERS

The group of polymers referred to as bioadhesive polymers is characterized by complex molecular structures composed of lengthy chains of monomers linked by covalent bonds. Their unique characteristics result from their specific architecture, which enables direct interactions with biological substrates. Many studies have emphasized the many benefits connected to these polymers. These advantages are varied and include the following: the extended retention of therapeutic agents at the application site, the delivery of drugs to specific anatomical sites, and the control of drug release kinetics for obtaining the best possible therapeutic results (K. Kumar et al. 2014; Shaikh et al. 2011; Carvalho et al. 2010).

The physicochemical properties of bioadhesive polymers differ from traditional polymers in addition to their functional advantages. Biomedical applications are ideally suited to them because of their viscoelastic nature, the presence of hydrogen-bonding functional groups, and their ability to swell and hydrate. They are also versatile and effective in a variety of biomedical conditions due to characteristics such as pH sensitivity, charge distribution along the structure of the polymer, molecule length, weight, and chain conformation (Shaikh et al. 2011).

The interaction of polymer chains with biological substrates is very similar to the mechanism of bioadhesive adhesion. First, the polymer chains are able to enter the substrate easier, and then noncovalent interactions occur. A variety of forces are involved in these interactions, including hydrogen bonding, hydrophobic interactions, Van der Waals forces, and electrostatic forces. Notably, the formation of hydrogen bonds is considerably facilitated by the presence of hydrophilic groups such as sulfate, amide, carboxyl, and hydroxyl groups within the polymer chains. This improves the adhesive interaction between the polymer chains and biological substrates (Shaikh et al. 2011).

Moreover, higher hydrogen bond-forming group concentrations are associated with improved polymer chain-substrate contact and stronger bioadhesive interactions. As a basis for the design and development of advanced drug delivery systems and medical devices, this complex chain of interactions emphasizes the adaptability and effectiveness of bioadhesive polymers in biomedical applications (K. Kumar et al. 2014; Shaikh et al. 2011).

Studies by Sudhakar et al. (2006) and Roy and Prabhakar (2010) indicate that a variety of characteristics are necessary for the safety and efficacy of bioadhesive polymers in biomedical applications (Sudhakar, Kuotsu, and Bandyopadhyay 2006; Roy and Prabhakar 2010). To provide accessibility for general use, these polymers should be, most importantly, widely available and economically viable. Apart from accessibility, safety concerns have precedence. To protect patient safety, polymers and the products of their degradation need to be subjected to an extensive examination to be certain they are non-toxic, non-irritating, and free of contaminants (K. Kumar et al. 2014).

Bioadhesive polymers must additionally include strong adhesive properties so they adhere to biological surfaces quickly and safely. This promotes the therapeutic compounds' efficient distribution and retention at the correct site. As important are the mechanical characteristics; polymers should be strong as well as resilient enough to tolerate physiological stresses and flexible enough to adapt to the mucosal surface (K. Kumar et al. 2014).

Bioadhesive polymers' performance is mostly determined by their physicochemical characteristics. Positive attributes including swelling capacity, spreadability, wettability, solubility, and biodegradability should be demonstrated. These characteristics affect the polymer's ability to interact with mucosal surfaces and release drugs in a controlled way (Shaikh et al. 2011; K. Kumar et al. 2014).

Moreover, bioadhesive polymers need to improve drug absorption via biological barriers in addition to facilitating drug release, thereby optimizing therapeutic results. To ensure consistent performance, stability in a range of environmental circumstances, such as hydrodynamic conditions and pH variations, is crucial (Shaikh et al. 2011).

Another essential characteristic is versatility; polymers need to have the ability to be used as bioadhesives in both liquid and solid phases, permitting a wide range of applications. In order to preserve polymer stability without reducing fluid characteristics, cross-linking is essential. However, to avoid reducing bond-forming groups, excessive cross-linking should be avoided (K. Kumar et al. 2014).

Comfort for the patient is crucial; bioadhesive polymers shouldn't irritate or inconvenience the patient, permitting them to continue about their regular activities without difficulties. To improve patient safety, they shouldn't promote the formation of secondary infections (K. Kumar et al. 2014; Saha et al. 2020).

In order to ensure efficacy, safety, and patient comfort the appropriate bioadhesive polymer must maintain these qualities. They provide an appropriate choice for improving therapeutic results in a range of biomedical applications due to their adaptability and compatibility with conventional drug delivery systems (L. Kumar et al. 2017; K. Kumar et al. 2014; Shaikh et al. 2011).

Bioadhesive polymer can be classified according to a variety of parameters, such as their charge (nonionic, cationic, and anionic) and origin (synthetic, semi-synthetic, or natural). However, the most detailed categorization depends on the chemical characteristics and properties of these polymers (K. Kumar et al. 2014; Shaikh et al. 2011; Khadem et al. 2022).

Polymers that included groups which generate bonds of covalent attraction, such as carboxylates, hydroxyls, and amino groups, define the first generation of bioadhesive polymers. These groups enable standard interactions with different surfaces. This group includes non-ionic polymers such as hydroxypropryl cellulose, anionic polymers such as those formed by acrylic acid, and cationic polymers such as chitosan (K. Kumar et al. 2014; Shaikh et al. 2011).

Conversely, the second generation of polymers are versatile polymers that can adhere to particular chemical structures on the surfaces of mucous membranes or cells. For example, some polymers have the ability to stick to lectins, which are proteins that identify sugar molecules on cell membranes and promote cytoadhesion (K. Kumar et al. 2014; de Lima et al. 2022; Yermak, Davydova, and Volod'ko 2022).

4.4.1 First Generation Bioadhesive Polymers (Non-Specific)

Anionic, cationic, and non-ionic polymers are the three categories of first-generation bioadhesive polymers (Carvalho et al. 2010). According to results found in Ludwing (2005), anionic and cationic bioadhesive polymers are particularly notable for their high bioadhesive properties (Ludwig 2005). This observation shows that importance of charge polymeric systems in improving bioadhesion and suggests an additional study of their mechanisms and applications is needed.

Anionic polymers interact strongly with positively charged sites on biological surfaces. They are identified by negatively charged functional groups such as carboxylates or sulfates. In this group, sodium alginates, sodium carboxymethylcellulose (NaCMC), and hyaluronic acid are significant examples of compounds that form strong connections with mucins, which are the main components of mucus (K. Kumar et al. 2014; Carvalho et al. 2010).

In contrast, positively charged functional groups such as amino groups are present in cationic polymers, which gives them the ability to interact electrostatically with mucosal surfaces that are negatively charged. Important examples are polyethyleneimine (PEI), poly-L-lysine, and chitosan, which are well known for their ability to adhere to mucins and offer significant bioadhesive properties (de Lima et al. 2022; K. Kumar et al. 2014; Ways, Lau, and Khutoryanskiy 2018).

The complex interaction between these charged polymers and biological surfaces play a crucial role in the generation of innovative biomedical formulations, such as bioadhesive patches and drug delivery systems. Researchers have to develop new strategies to improve therapeutic interventions and biomedical products aimed at improving treatment by bioadhesive with the advantages of the properties of anionic and cationic polymers (K. Kumar et al. 2014; L. Kumar et al. 2017; de Lima et al. 2022).

4.4.1.1 Anionic Polymers

Anionic polymers are widely used in pharmaceuticals formulations due to their low toxicity and high bioadhesive potential. They usually have sulfate and carboxyl groups, which show negative charges at pH values greater than their pKa in the environment. Polycarbophil, sodium alginate, sodium carboxymethylcellulose (NaCMC), poly(acrylic acid) derivates, and poly[(maleic acid)-co-(vinyl methyl ether)] are a few anionic polymer examples (de Lima et al. 2022; K. Kumar et al. 2014).

Many studies have been conducted on polymeric derivatives derived from poly(acrylic acid), such as polycarbophil and cabomers, as mucoadhesive platforms for gastrointestinal tract medications administration. Insoluble in aqueous solutions, polycarbophil has a significant capacity to swell at neutral pH levels, allowing for significant tangling in the mucus layer. Its capacity to change mass by up to 100 times in aqueous solutions with a neutral pH emphasizes its potential for mucoadhesion (de Lima et al. 2022; Ways, Lau, and Khutoryanskiy 2018; Carvalho et al. 2010). Furthermore, polycarbophil's non-ionized carboxylic acid groups adhere directly to mucosal surfaces via hydrogen bonding interactions. With characteristics such as non-toxicity and non-irritability, and Food and Drug Administration approval for safe oral use, polycarbophil polymers, which can be found in a range of molecular weights, produce transparent and flexible gel networks. It is generally know that the electrostatic repulsion between anionic groups promotes the gel formation (de Lima et al. 2022; Carvalho et al. 2010; K. Kumar et al. 2014). Additionally, differences in cross-linking agents and amounts have been demonstrated between carbomer and polycarbophil. Polycarbophil polymers use divinyl glycol as a cross-linking agent, while carbomers use allyl sucrose or allyl pentaerythritol (K. Kumar et al. 2014).

Since their introduction and patent in 1957, carbomers have attracted attention from a range of industries due to their variety of applications. These polymers are mostly used as thickening agents in drug delivery systems, but also have bioadhesive properties and are utilized as a flow behavior modifier for polymer dispersion. Carbomers are a family of synthetic polymeric materials with high molecular weights. They are made of acrylic acid that has been cross-linked by a chain of allyl sucrose or allyl ethers of pentaerythritol, for example (de Lima et al. 2022).

Carbomers are a white and light powder, with an acidic flavor. They are hygroscopic, so when they come into contact with water they expand significantly, increasing up to 1000 times in volume and 10 times in size. With chain ionization, the carboxyl groups present in the acrylic acid chain are crucial for gel formation, and the neutralization causes negatively charged groups to be electrostatically repelled, which promotes gel formation and drug retention (de Lima et al. 2022).

Carbomers are widely known for their bioadhesive qualities. They can hydrate, expand, and absorb water without losing their cross-linked structure. Their use for a variety of biomedical applications is facilitated by their insolubility in water. The primary mechanism of mucoadhesion is the formation of hydrogen bonds between the sialic acid groups of mucin glycoproteins and the carboxylic acid groups of carbomers (Smart 2005).

Several routes of administration, including topical, nasal, oral, ophthalmic, vaginal, intestinal, and rectal, are useful for bioadhesive formulations that contain carbomers. Numerous studies have shown that carbomers are low in toxicity and have a low probability of causing irritation, which makes them a popular choice for bioadhesive applications (Smart 2005).

Neutralized carbomers, which have a pH level between 4 an 6, offer several benefits, including safety, bioavailability, protection against enzymes, compatibility with a wide range of active ingredients, compatibility with different forms of bonding, thermal stability, and favorable organoleptic properties. Their popularity and effectiveness in pharmaceutical formulations are amplified by several regulatory agencies' approval of them (Smart 2005).

Additionally, carbomers contain several categories that are differentiated by the degree of cross-linking and manufacturing conditions, each with a distinct relevance and applicability for a range of pharmaceutical formulations. The carbomers 934P, 971P, and 974P are examples and are designated with a "P" to denote pharmaceutical grades that are appropriate for oral administration as they have a minimal residual benzene concentration.

The cellulose derivatives polymers have the intrinsic property of absorbing water from mucus, adding to their adhesive qualities, which are important for a variety of biomedical applications. The most prevalent organic chemical in the world, cellulose, is mostly derived from plants and has a wide range of mechanical and pharmacological properties due to differences in the size, shape, and degree of crystallinity of its particles. A wide range of semi-synthetic derivatives, such as cellulose ethers and cellulose esters, are also present in cellulose. Some well-known examples that are used in bioadhesive prepatations are sodium carboxymethyl cellulose, hydroxyethyl cellulose, hydroxypropyl cellulose, methylcellulose, carboxymethyl cellulose, and hydroxypropymethyl cellulose (Seddiqi et al. 2021; de Lima et al. 2022).

Furthermore, the adaptability of cellulose derivatives makes it easier to incorporate them into formulations for bioadhesives, where they are essential for improving mucoadhesive properties. This emphasizes the importance of cellulose and its derivatives in the context of bioadhesive technology, providing options for the development of biomedical devices and advanced drug delivery systems (Oprea and Voicu 2020; Seddiqi et al. 2021).

Moreover, anionic polymers have a variety of versatile applications in bioadhesive formulations, which not only highlights their significance in drug delivery, but also opens up new possibilities for pharmaceutical science and technology to explore in terms of optimization and innovation.

4.4.1.2 Cationic Polymers

Among cationic polymers, chitosan is one of the most researched. Formed from the deacetylation of chitin, which is the second most prevalent polysaccharide in the world, chitosan exhibits an abundance of interesting characteristics with uses in multiple sectors including industrial, pharmaceutical, and agricultural. Its use as a metal-recovering agent in industry, an antipathogenic agent in agriculture, and a film-forming material in cosmetics demonstrate how adaptable it is. Chitosan is also used in the production of paper, as a hypolipidemic dietary component, and as a dye-binder for textiles (Desai et al. 2023).

Among the range of bioadhesive polymers being studied, chitosan is well-known because of its great toxicological profile, biodegradability, and biocompatibility. In contrast to polycarbophil, which mainly attaches to mucus by hydrogen bonding, chitosan is recognized for its ability to connect through ionic interactions between its principal amino functional groups and the mucus's sialic and sulphonic acid substructures. In addition, chitosan's amino and hydroxyl groups enable hydrogen-bonding interactions with mucus, and the molecules' linear shape provides enough chain flexibility for efficient interpenetration (de Lima et al. 2022; Kaur and Singh 2020; Desai et al. 2023).

Chitosan can improve drug absorption through the paracellular pathway by neutralizing fixed anionic sites in the tightly bound connections between mucosal cells, in addition to its capability to improve drug delivery through a mucoadhesive mechanism. Interestingly, chitosan becomes more soluble in aqueous acidic environments as the degree of deacetylation increases, whereas chitin becomes soluble at a deacetylation level of more than 50%. The protonation of the $-NH_2$ function on the C-2 position of the D-glucosamine repeat unit is responsible for this increased solubility (Desai et al. 2023; Shahid et al. 2020).

The main advantage of using chitosan in pharmaceutical applications is that it may be chemically modified, especially at the C-2 position, which allows for the synthesis of new polymers with additional functionality. These alterations permit chitosan's characteristics to be modified for certain pharmacological and technical applications (Cheung et al. 2015; Kedir et al. 2022).

4.4.2 Second-Generation Bioadhesion Polymers (Specific)

Using conventional non-specific (first generation) bioadhesive systems has a significant disadvantage: adhesion can occur at unexpected places. Non-specific polymers occasionally connect to locations that are not the intended target, a process known as off-target binding, making them less effective. Moreover, mucus turnover rates greatly affect non-specific polymers, and a higher turnover rate reduces the effectiveness of bioadhesion. So, second-generation polymer platforms that are less susceptible to mucus turnover rates are more desirable, with this phenomenon described as "cytoadhesion." Some of these species also bind to mucosal surfaces (Kaur and Singh 2020; de Lima et al. 2022).

This new generation-specific bioadhesive polymers shows no dependence on mucus turnover rates and efficiently target mucus surfaces according to protein and carbohydrate composition. Changing from non-specific bioadhesive platforms to second-generation bioadhesive polymers has the potential to improve the precision and efficacy of targeted drug delivery systems (Smart 2004; K. Kumar et al. 2014; Lehr 2000).

4.4.2.1 Lectins

Lectins, naturally occurring proteins, have an essential role in biological recognition that involves cells and proteins. Lectins are important proteins in pathophysiological processes because certain bacteria use them to adhere to cells during infection. The use of specific cytoadhesives, such as lectins, show promise in the context of improving mucosal delivery (Santos et al. 2014; Gavrovic-Jankulovic and Prodanovic 2011; Neutsch et al. 2011).

Lectins are a structurally diverse class of proteins and glycoproteins that are, impressively, capable of reversibly adhering to carbohydrate residues. After lectins first stick to mucosal cells, they can stay on the cell surface or adhere to the cells by receptor-mediated adhesion, which result in absorption through endocytosis. Because of that, lectin-based platforms promoting drug absorption mediated controlled drug delivery, while also facilitating targeted specific adherence. So, lectin-mediated drug delivery systems are able to transfer the drug from the mucus layer to the cell layer, offering an initial and reversible interaction (Lehr 2000).

However, the effects of prolonged lectin administration are still unclear, and many lectins demonstrate toxicity or immunogenicity. Additionally, lectin-induced antibodies may block future contact between the mucosal epithelial cells surfaces and lectin-based delivery systems (Lavelle et al. 2004, 2000).

In bioadhesive platforms, lectin-based polymers such as peanut agglutinin, ulex europaeus agglutinin, and lentil lectin are utilized. These polymers enable controlled distribution of bioactive compounds through active cell-mediated uptake mechanisms and targeted bioadhesion. Due to their reversible adhesion, lectins, compared to first-generation polymers, are not prematurely inactivated by mucus shed, which facilitates the high dissemination of lectin-based delivery systems. However, despite their benefits, lectins may present immunological and toxicological problems, such as the potential for lectin-induced antibodies to make patients more vulnerable to systemic anaphylaxis after further exposure (Lehr 2000; Lavelle et al. 2004).

4.4.2.2 Thiolated Polymers

Hydrophilic polymers such as polycrylates, chitosan, or deacetylated gellan gum are the precursors of thiolated polymers. Thiol groups, added into these polymers through thiolation, are essential for improving their mucoadhesive properties. The presence of thiol groups facilitates the formation of covalent bonds with mucus gel layer's cysteine. Similar to the natural mechanism of released mucus glycoproteins, which are likewise covalently fixed in the mucus layer through disulfide bonds, this covalent anchoring mechanism increases the residence time and enhances bioavailability (Puri et al. 2020; Younas et al. 2023).

Thiolated polymers have better bioadhesive qualities than first-generation platforms, mainly because of non-covalent secondary interactions. Because of their intrinsic covalent bonding processes, second-generation systems are less vulnerable to pH imbalance or ionic strength variations. In contrast to first-generation polymers, which show anomalous transport of active pharmaceutical ingredients into bulk solution, thiolated polymers usually exhibit a diffusion-controlled drug release mechanism (Carvalho et al. 2010; Puri et al. 2020; Bernkop-Schnürch, Schwarz, and Steininger 1999).

Thiolated polymers contain numerous hydrophilic polymer derivatives, including polyacrylates and chitosan. Thioglycolic acid, chitosan–thioethylamidine, poly(acrylic acid)–cysteine, and alginate–cysteine are some of the most common examples of thiolated polymers. Through covalent interactions with cysteine-rich areas of the mucus layer, the insertion of thiol groups inside these polymers improves residence duration and bioavailability. Furthermore, thiolated polymers can form disulfide bonds and become covalently fixed in the mucus layer, which further improves their bioadhesive qualities and influences the drug release process (Bernkop-Schnürch, Schwarz, and Steininger 1999; Federer, Kurpiers, and Bernkop-Schnürch 2021; Younas et al. 2023; Puri et al. 2020).

Overall, thiolated polymers offer good adhesive qualities, extended residence times, and controlled drug release with better therapeutic results in a range of biomedical applications. So, they are potential polymers in bioadhesive technology.

4.4.3 NATURAL BIOADHESIVE POLYMERS

Natural bioadhesive polymers are composed of a variety of substances, mostly polysaccharides including starch, guar gum, cantham gum, gellan gum, and carrageenan. These polymers are useful in drug delivery systems and biological applications because they have intrinsic bioadhesive qualities, similar to glycosaminoglycans and natural peptides such as gelatin (Huang et al. 2024; Ke et al. 2020).

Derived from guar beans, guar gum is unique among galactomannans that have been certified safe by regulatory agencies. Some of its derivates, including hydrocypropyl guar, have demonstrated potential as bioadhesive polymers. The negatively charged polysaccharide xanthan gum, which is generated by bacteria, has also been used in ophthalmic formulations because of its gel-forming properties (Yuan et al. 2019; Froelich et al. 2023).

The synergistic rheological and bioadhesive capabilities of guar gum and chitosan, another bioadhesive polymer, have been demonstrated, especially in ophthalmic formulations (Yuan et al. 2019).

Pectin, an anionic polysaccharide derived from plant cell walls, has thickening characteristics and promotes bioadhesive interactions by combining mucin and pectin, for example. Prolonged residence times are the consequence of this interaction, especially in applications involving the oral mucosa (Laurén et al. 2018; Martau, Mihai, and Vodnar 2019; Thirawong, Kennedy, and Sriamornsak 2008; Klemetsrud et al. 2013).

Hyaluronic acid is particularly notable for its mucoadhesive and biocompatibility. Hyaluronic acid improves the mucoadhesive qualities of pectin gels when combined with fructooligosaccharides and low methylester pectin, indicating potential for vaginal applications (Laurén et al. 2018; Martau, Mihai, and Vodnar 2019).

More mucoadhesive forces are present in gellan gum and its derivative carboxymethyl gellan gum than in gellan gum alone. These bacterial-produced polysaccharides have been thoroughly researched for a range of uses, such as regenerative medicine and formulations for the nasal and ocular cavities (Jelkmann et al. 2020).

Carrageenans are derived from edible seaweeds and are useful in medicinal formulations because of their thickening, bioadhesive, and gelling properties. Because of its strong bioadhesive qualities, tragacanth, a plant derived from *Astragalus*, exhibits promise as an excipient in drug delivery systems (Prajapati and Patel 2024; Kali et al. 2023).

The mucoadhesive properties of gelatin, a naturally occurring polypeptide produced from collagen, and polysaccharides from *Bletilla striata* have also been studied and provide opportunities for a variety of biological and drug delivery applications (Ji et al. 2020; Thacker et al. 2020).

4.4 INFLUENCE OF POLYMER PROPERTIES ON BIOADHESION

Within the context of bioadhesion theories, the characteristics of polymers are crucial in establishing the probability and degree of contact between polymers and biological surfaces. These characteristics include both functional and structural elements that together affect how adhesively polymers interact with biological surfaces (Roy and Prabhakar 2010; K. Kumar et al. 2014).

The chemical structure of polymers, which includes their molecular weight, chain length, and branching, is an important factor to take into consideration. Due to more chances for molecular interaction with mucin molecules, polymers with longer chains and higher molecular weights typically show stronger mucoadhesive potential. Similarly, by adding more points of contact with mucous surfaces, expanding within polymer structures can improve their adhesive properties (Roy et al. 2009; Bayer 2022).

Additionally, polymer chains' functional groups have an important effect on bioadhesion. It has been observed that hydrophilic groups, such as hydroxyl, carboxyl, and amine groups, contribute to further increase adherence (Pham et al. 2021).

Moreover, the bioadhesive behavior of polymers can be influenced by their physicochemical characteristics, which include their flexibility, swelling capacity, and hydrophobicity/hydrophilicity balance. Better bioadhesion is demonstrated by polymers that have an appropriate ratio of hydrophilic to hydrophobic molecules, which optimizes interactions with the complex mucosal environment. Furthermore, flexible polymer chains improve contact and adherence by adjusting more effectively to the atypicality of biological surfaces (Pham et al. 2021).

The potential to modify or control these polymer properties provides an opportunity for personalized bioadhesive delivery system design. Through alternations of parameters such as molecular weight, branching, functional group composition, and physicochemical properties, the adhesive behavior of polymers can be customized to satisfy the requirements for specific applications. The study of mucosal drug delivery has been advanced by this specific approach, resulting in its potential to develop mucoadhesive delivery systems with improved efficacy, biocompatibility, and drug release behaviors (Shaikh et al. 2011; Carvalho et al. 2010).

4.4.4 Contribution of Functional Groups

Bioadhesive polymers adhere and connect to biological substrates mainly through interpenetration, which is followed by the formation of secondary non-covalent bonds. These connections, which are mostly formed by hydrogen bonding, are essential for improving the binding between the substrate and the polymer. For the purpose of creating specific drug delivery platforms, bioadhesive polymers with hydrophilic functional groups, such as carboxyl (COOH), hydroxyl (OH), amide (NH2), and sulfate (SO4H) groups, are especially advantageous (Shaikh et al. 2011; K.Kumar et al. 2014; de Lima et al. 2022).

Mucin glycoproteins and polymers form a strong network through secondary contacts and physical entanglements, especially hydrogen bonds. Mucin glycoproteins bind more strongly with polymers that have a high density of accessible hydrogen bonding groups, which improves the mucoadhesive properties of the glycoproteins. These mucoadhesive polymers usually promote interactions via secondary chemical bonds in addition to physical entanglements. As a result, strongly cross-linked networks are created, which increase the polymer's adhesive bond with the mucosal surface significantly (de Lima et al. 2022; K. Kumar et al. 2014; Shaikh et al. 2011).

Carbohydrate groups in mucins are important sites for mucoadhesive contacts, where hydrophobic bonding, especially with fucose groups, or electrostatic interactions are important. Hagesaether and Sande's recent research, among others, focused attention on the significance of hydrogen bonding in mucoadhesion process (Hagesaether and Sande 2007). For example, the mucoadhesiveness of different mucus/pectin samples is dramatically reduced after the addition of urea, a well-know disruptor of hydrogen bonds. This disruption highlights the crucial function that hydrogen bonding plays in mucoadhesive contacts by causing a decrease in cohesion and a loss of synergy within the combined pectin/mucin combination (Pham et al. 2021).

Understanding these complicated processes provides important knowledge for the development and improvement of bioadhesive drug delivery systems that exhibit increased specificity and efficacy. Bioadhesive formulations can be customized by researchers for specific and prolonged drug delivery applications by changing the characteristics of polymers to optimize hydrogen bonding and interactions between functional groups.

4.4.5 LEVEL OF HYDRATION

The level of hydration has an influence on the bioadhesive strength of polymeric components in drug delivery systems, which is an important consideration. Many polymers can still have adhesive properties in circumstances where there is an abundance of water. Osmotic forces and capillary attraction between the wet biological surface and the dry polymer interact to result in this phenomenon. These forces help to promote adhesion by thickening and dehydrating the mucus layer (Shaikh et al. 2011; Del Grosso et al. 2020).

That form of adhesion must be different from "wet-on-wet" adhesion, which occurs when swelling mucoadhesive polymers adhere to mucosal surfaces. Although hydration is necessary for the polymer chains to relax and interpenetrate, excessive hydration can cause a slippery mucilage formation, which can reduce mucoadhesion and retention. This distinction depends on attention to the intricate relationship between the dynamics of mucoadhesion and hydration (Del Grosso et al. 2020).

When referring to extended bioadhesive effects, cross-linked polymers which restrict hydration to a certain degree may be advantageous. Researchers can modify bioadhesive formulations to attain specific adhesion and retention characteristics by changing the degree of hydration. This comprehensive understanding of hydration dynamics emphasizes how tailored strategies are crucial to developing mucoadhesive drug delivery systems for a range of biological applications (Shaikh et al. 2011; Vigani et al. 2023).

Additional research on the processes for hydration-dependent adhesion is necessary considering the complex nature of hydration's effects on bioadhesion. Through an explanation of these mechanisms, researchers could propose innovative methods that improve the efficacy and adaptability of bioadhesion drug delivery systems, so enhancing the patient experience in treatments.

4.4.6 POLYMER MOLECULAR WEIGHT, CROSS-LINKING STRENGTH, CHAIN LENGTH, AND CONFORMATION

The impact of structural polymeric characteristics on bioadhesion, including factors such as diffusion, entanglement, and molecular weight, is a complex, and currently crucial, topic of drug delivery research. Molecular weight in particular has been demonstrated to be a significant factor in determining how polymers' bioadhesive characteristics are developed. Although a high molecular weight is necessary to promote entanglement, it is crucial to remember that excessively long polymer chains may eventually become more difficult to diffuse and interpenetrate biological surfaces. As a result, determining the ideal molecular weight for bioadhesion is still difficult because polymeric systems are too distinct from each other for an accepted norm to be established (Roy and Prabhakar 2010; Peppas, Thomas, and McGinity 2011; Kumar et al. 2017; Singh and Sharma 2014).

Moreover, the degree of cross-linking present in a polymer system has a significant impact on the bioadhesive behavior of the system. For example, cross-linked hydrophilic polymers tend to swell when exposed to water, which helps to maintain their structural integrity. On the other hand, linear hydrophilic polymers with similar high molecular weights typically expand and dissolve. This swelling phenomenon is important for bioadhesion because it increases the surface area accessible for mucus interpenetration, for example, and allows for improved control over drug release (K. Kumar et al. 2014; Shaikh et al. 2011).

However, when the cross-link density increases, there is an apparent reduction in chain mobility, which reduces the bioadhesive strength because there is a decreased effective chain length that can penetrate the mucus layer. Another important factor in promoting entanglement and interpenetration inside the mucosal gel matrix, for example, is chain flexibility. Stronger mucoadhesive contacts are produced by increased chain mobility, which facilitates higher degrees of polymer inter-diffusion and interpenetration within the complex mucus network (Bayer 2022; Roy et al. 2009).

To summarize, an extensive knowledge of the complex interactions between polymer structure, molecular weight, cross-linking, and chain flexibility is an essential precondition for developing bioadhesive formulations that are optimized. Through careful analysis and manipulation of these complex interactions, researchers can attempt to develop personalized drug delivery systems with enhanced bioadhesive capabilities, prepared for use with the wide range of biological obstacles present in current therapeutic circumstances.

4.4.7 ELECTRICAL CHARGE AND pH

The bioadhesion of polymers is significantly influenced by their charge density. For bioadhesion and toxicity reasons, polyanions are frequently preferred over polycations. The pH level of the physiological environment has a significant impact on this charge density due to the impacts the dissociation of functional groups within polymers. In particular, polymers and mucus have a great deal of potential for hydrogen bonding, especially when the polymers have undissociated anionic chain functional groups (L. Kumar et al. 2017; Cencer et al. 2014).

For carboxylated polymers, it is considered that maintaining pH levels below the corresponding pKa value promotes bioadhesion more effectively (L. Kumar et al. 2017). According to a study by Park and Robinson, successful bioadhesion in polyacrylic acid systems requires about 80% protonation of carboxyl groups (Park and Robinson 1987). A further study by Sudhakar et al. suggests that carboxylic groups in polyacrylic acids are only effective as interaction sites when they are in their acidic form (Sudhakar, Kuotsu, and Bandyopadhyay 2006).

Although bioadhesion processes are optimized in low pH conditions, it is important to highlight that bioadhesion may not be completely affected at higher pH values. A modification in spatial conformation from a helical to a rod-like structure is caused by the repulsion of homologous -COO⁻ functional groups at elevated pH levels. By causing these functional groups to be more accessible for inter-diffusion and interpenetration, the modification improves bioadhesive interactions (Roy and Prabhakar 2010; Cencer et al. 2014; Bu and Pandit 2022).

Furthermore, as can be observed in ionized polyacrylic acid systems, a charge that is not positive may cause anionic species to become repulsed over the pKa of mucin. During these circumstances, negatively charged mucins and positively charged polymers, such as chitosan, can create polyelectrolyte complexes that provide strong mucoadhesion (Shaikh et al. 2011; Lankalapalli and Kolapalli 2009; Lu 2018).

Anionic, cationic, and non-ionic systems are the three basic classes of bioadhesive polymers that can be distinguished by absolute charge. Of them, anionic polymer systems, such as polyacrylic acids, are widely used in medicinal applications. Studies involving the attachment of different chemical entities to chitosan have clearly proven the influence of polymer charge on bioadhesion. The addition of anionic functional groups, such as ethylene diamine tetra acetic acid (EDTA), significantly improved mucoadhesive capacity, but cationic chitosan demonstrated substantial adhesiveness when compared to the control. It's interesting to note that systems with both cationic and anionic characteristics, such as a diethylenetriaminepentaacetic acid (DTPA)–chitosan complex, showed reduced mucoadhesive strength, which was explained by a decrease in total charge density. This demonstrates the complex interactions between polymer charge and bioadhesive characteristics, emphasizing how crucial it is to understand and optimize these interactions to develop bioadhesive drug delivery systems that are effective (Roy and Prabhakar 2010; Nafee et al. 2004).

4.4.8 POLYMER CONCENTRATION

The concentration of polymers has an essential function in determining the bioadhesive strength and has an important influence on the efficiency of drug delivery systems. The influence of polymer concentration changes with the delivery system's physical state; solid-state and semisolid-state formulations require different considerations (L.Kumar et al. 2017; Shaikh et al. 2011; Roy and Prabhakar 2010; K. Kumar et al. 2014).

There is an ideal polymer concentration for each individual polymer in semisolid formulations, such as gels or ointments. An observed decrease in adhesion strength occurs beyond this ideal concentration. The reduced availability of polymer chains for mucus layer interpenetration is the cause of this occurrence. The extra polymer might inhibit against improve mucoadhesion once the concentration exceeds over the ideal limit (Araújo et al. 2022; Shaikh et al. 2011).

In contrast, the association between polymer concentration and bioadhesive strength changes in solid dose forms, such as buccal tablets or patches. An increase in polymer concentration in these formulations usually results in an increase in adhesive strength. More binding points for interaction with the mucus layer are made possible by higher concentrations of mucoadhesive polymer, for example, which results in improved adherence and longer residence times at the application site (Shaikh et al. 2011; K. Kumar et al. 2014; Amorós-Galicia et al. 2022).

Recognizing the intricate correlation between polymer concentration and bioadhesive strength is crucial for the development and improvement of successful drug delivery systems. Researchers can optimize the therapeutic efficacy and patient compliance of bioadhesive formulations by carefully determining the right concentration of bioadhesive polymer depending on specific characteristics of the delivery system and target tissue (Roy and Prabhakar 2010; Shaikh et al. 2011; L. Kumar et al. 2017).

4.5   MUCU-PERMEATION SYSTEMS

When it comes to oral administration, medication delivery systems have biological limitations. The gastrointestinal system is a key barrier because it is covered in mucus, which acts as a protective barrier against foreign particles. The mucus layer is a viscous aqueous gel made up of water (~95%) and glycoprotein macromolecules (mucins). The thickness ranges from 5 to 500 μm, with an average of 80 μm, and fluctuates throughout the gastrointestinal system. While the duodenum has a continuous mucus layer, the small and large intestines have discontinuous layers (Tarabova et al. 2016; Grondin et al. 2020; Song et al. 2023; Miyazaki, Sasaki, and Mizuuchi 2023).

These mucus layer properties present obstacles for drug absorption. Prolonged interactions with the mucosa, whether caused by steric impediments or adhesion processes, might reduce drug absorption in the body (Figure 4.2). Excessively strong bioadhesive forces for prolonged periods of time may impede drug absorption, even though mucoadhesive systems are intended to adhere to the mucosa to improve drug delivery (Figure 4.2). Therefore, to maintain efficient absorption while reducing unwanted interactions with the mucosa, drug delivery systems must balance mucoadhesion and mucopermeability (Subramanian, Langer, and Traverso 2022; Barmpatsalou 2023).

4.5.1   STRATEGIES FOR MUCUS-PERMEATION

Strategies for breaking the mucus gel layer's barrier are critical for successful medication administration; however, typical procedures that involve the breakdown of the mucus gel layer raise major toxicological concerns due to its protective function. As a result, recent research has focused on nanocarrier systems that can pierce the mucus barrier without causing significant damage (Yan and Sha 2023; Sato et al. 2023).

These nanocarrier systems can be divided into two categories: passive and active. Passive methods aim to reduce particle-mucus interactions. Promising options include particles with slippery surfaces and self-nanoemulsifying drug delivery systems (SNEDDS). Active systems, on the other hand, interact with mucus to promote particle permeability, frequently using disulfide bridge-breaking agents and proteolytic enzymes (Sato et al. 2023).

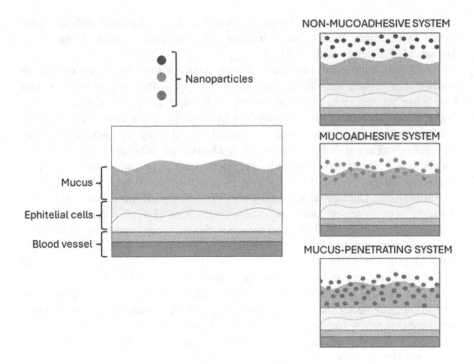

FIGURE 4.2   Representation of nanoparticle systems with mucoadhesiveness and mucus-permeation.

Furthermore, solutions for preventing particles from diffusing out of the mucus gel layer have been developed, with a focus on thiomers and zeta potential modification systems.

4.5.1.1   Slippery Surface Strategy

Many viruses spread quickly via a mucus layer similar to water. Their surfaces are extensively coated with positive and negative charged groups, resulting in a net neutral surface. This high surface charge density most likely promotes a hydrophilic surface, reducing hydrophobic interactions between a mucus and a virus trapped in the mucous layer. Thus, a balanced density of positive and negative surface charges may improve particle movement through mucus by reducing electrostatic interactions (Boegh and Nielsen 2015; Subramanian, Langer, and Traverso 2022).

Certain viruses, such as poliovirus and human papillomavirus, exploit this strategy as their surfaces are neutral and inert to mucus. These viruses have a densely charged envelope, both positively and negatively, which results in a final neutral charge. This structure allows them to avoid potential electrostatic interactions and/or hydrogen bonds with mucus components (Subramanian, Langer, and Traverso 2022; Boegh and Nielsen 2015; Wallace et al. 2021).

Based on this principle, combining high charge density anionic and cationic polymers can result in "slippery" nanoparticulate systems. Polyelectrolyte complexes

created by mixing oppositely charged polymers have shown greater diffusion efficiency in intestinal mucus than individual polymers (Subramanian, Langer, and
Traverso 2022; Cortés et al. 2021).

As a result, nano/micro carriers in delivery systems with electrically uncharged
surfaces can remain inert to the mucosa if they are sufficiently hydrophilic and
have a low propensity to hydrogen binding with mucus components. Recently, two
major methodologies for constructing such systems have been developed. The first
involves combining polymers with opposing electrical charges to produce particles
with densely charged, but neutral, surfaces. The second technique involves coating
carriers with neutral and hydrophilic polymers, such as polyethyleneglycol (PEG)
(Sato et al. 2023).

Furthermore, nanoparticles coated with a PEG of specific molecular weights and
densities have increased mucus penetrating capacities. Several studies have demonstrated the efficacy of PEGylated nanoparticles in penetrating mucosal barriers,
indicating potential possibilities for therapeutic peptide administration (Xu et al.
2015; Maisel et al. 2016).

Surface chemistry is important in the mucus permeation behavior of nanoparticles. For example, unmodified polystyrene nanoparticles only partially penetrated
human cervical mucus, but carboxyl-modified polystyrene nanoparticles of the same
size were completely trapped in the mucus gel layer (Inchaurraga et al. 2015; Schmid
et al. 2023; Wright et al. 2022). These results emphasize the importance of surface
characteristics in nanoparticle interactions with mucus.

4.5.1.2 SNEDDS Strategy

Self-emulsifying systems at the nanometric scale are a viable technique for improving intestinal mucosal permeability. When coupled with water, SNEDDS create an
O/W nanoemulsion from oil, surfactant, and cosurfactant. These nanodroplets have a
hydrophobic surface, which reduces interactions with the mucus layer. Furthermore,
their modest size, typically about 650 nm, along with their capacity to deform, allows
for diffusion through mucus gel layers with different particle sizes (Sato et al. 2023;
Eid, Elmarzugi, and Jaradat 2019; Mahajan et al. 2024).

Arshad and colleagues investigated the diffusion of several fluorescently labeled
SNEDDS formulations through intestinal mucus layers (Arshad et al. 2022). The
findings revealed that the mucus permeability of these formulations was size-depen-
dent, with smaller droplets having higher penetration rates. For example, formulations with droplet diameters of 12 nm demonstrated 70.3% penetration, but those
with diameters of 455.5 nm showed just 8.3% permeation. Furthermore, the composition of formulation excipients was discovered to influence SNEDDS penetration through mucus, with some excipients, such as Cremophor RH 40 and triacetin,
exhibiting promising capabilities for enhancing mucus permeability (Arshad et al.
2022).

In another study, SNEDDS formulations with equal droplet sizes were created, and
it was discovered that a single excipient alteration might considerably affect mucus
permeability. For example, substituting Labrafil M1944CS for Lauroglycol FCC as
the oil, combined with adjusting the oil/surfactant/cosurfactant ratios, resulted in a

significant improvement in permeability from 25% to 50% (Subramanian, Langer, and Traverso 2022; Wright et al. 2022).

Furthermore, modified surface SNEDDS formulations were developed by combining surfactants with positively or negatively charged functional groups. The inclusion of cationic surfactants resulted in larger droplet sizes and decreased mucus permeability, but the combination of anionic and cationic surfactants enhanced permeability when compared to the unmodified formulation.

4.5.1.3   Disulfide Breaking Strategy

Numerous studies have demonstrated the effectiveness of mucolytic medicines, such as N-acetylcysteine, in bypassing the substantial barrier created by mucus gel. Their efficacy is based on the breaking down of disulfide connections within mucin fibers, which reduces the viscosity of the mucus matrix (Subramanian, Langer, and Traverso 2022; Yan and Sha 2023; Sato et al. 2023).

Recent studies focus on the production of nanoparticles that can release mucolytic chemicals in a regulated manner while passing through the mucus layer without causing significant damage. Controlled release techniques, inspired by certain bacteria's capacity to traverse through mucus via mucolytic enzyme secretion, attempts to provide mucolytic system. Sulfhydryl substances such as reduced glutathione, dithiothreitol, 4-mercaptobenzoic acid, N-acetylcysteine, and cysteine are among the most promising mucolytic components because they facilitate the breakage of disulfide bonds inside the mucus gel barrier. These compounds can be integrated into nanocarriers with drugs, providing a possible route for improving drug delivery via mucus barriers while maintaining structural integrity and protective function (Yan and Sha 2023; Sato et al. 2023; Subramanian, Langer, and Traverso 2022).

4.5.1.4   Proteolytic Enzyme Strategy

The immobilization of mucolytic enzymes, such as trypsin, papain, and bromelain, on the surface of polymer nanoparticles is a potential technique for breaking down the mucus barrier. These enzymes have the ability to break the cross-linked networks of mucus glycoproteins, functioning as mucolytic agents and allowing for localized disruption of the mucus layer. Enzymes can be immobilized on polymer nanoparticles surfaces using a variety of methods, including covalent bonding with or without spacers and ionic interactions (Zhu et al. 2022).

Müller and collaborators investigated the efficacy of proteolytic enzyme-modified nanoparticles as mucus-penetrant delivery vehicles (Müller et al. 2014). Their results demonstrated that the mucolytic activity of these modified nanocarriers greatly increased particle transport rates while decreasing the viscoelastic characteristics of pig intestinal mucus when compared to unmodified particles. Papain-functionalized nanoparticles showed promise in terms of penetrating the mucosal barrier and avoiding fast mucus clearance. These proteolytic enzyme-functionalized nanocarriers demonstrated the ability to cross the mucus layer, infiltrate deeper mucus regions, and concentrate significantly in the duodenum and jejunum, which have the most surface area within the small intestine (Müller et al. 2014).

Moreover, Samaridou and colleagues created surface-functionalized PLGA nanoparticles with proteolytic enzymes, including trypsin, papain, and bromelain, utilizing a two-step carbodiimide conjugation (Samaridou et al. 2014). Functionalized nanoparticles have greater permeability in pig intestinal mucus than non-functionalized ones. Papain- and bromelain-conjugated nanoparticles showed increased permeability rates, implying that they could improve nanoparticle penetration in mucus gel (Samaridou et al. 2014).

Drug integration into nanoparticles can occur before or after the immobilization of proteolytic enzymes on their surface. Drug-loaded polymeric nanoparticles coupled with enzymes can be prepared using a variety of processes, including ionic gelation and double emulsion. It is worth emphasizing that alternate enzymes, such as glycosidases, should be explored when adding therapeutic peptides to avoid proteolytic degradation (Samaridou et al. 2014).

While enzyme-coupled nanocarrier technology is still in its early stages, research has predominantly used polymers as carrier matrices, including poly(acrylic acid) (PAA) and poly(lactic-co-glycolic acid) (PLGA). However, significant research into a varied spectrum of polymers with varying characteristics is expected over the following years (Samaridou et al. 2014; Tewari et al. 2022; Das et al. 2020).

4.5.2 MUCUS-PERMEATION POLYMERS

Overcoming the mucus barrier is an important part of developing effective drug delivery systems, and mucoadhesive polymers are frequently used to extend the retention duration of pharmacological dosage forms on mucosal surfaces. These polymers increase adhesion by a variety of interactions, including electrostatic forces, chain entanglement, and van der Waals forces. An alternate strategy would be to design systems that can efficiently penetrate the mucus barrier and concentrate near the epithelial surface. Combining both adhesion and penetration effects is a potential method for oral drug delivery systems, allowing for an extended residence time close to the cell membrane (Sandri et al. 2015; Roy et al. 2009).

In recent years, there has been a focus on developing dosage forms with both mucoadhesive and mucus-permeating properties. This approach aims to maximize the benefits of both strategies in overcoming the mucus barrier. Particularly, the utilization of mucus-penetrating properties has been predominantly observed in the development of nanoparticulate systems. The physicochemical characteristics of nanoparticles, including size, charge, hydrophobicity, and surface properties, play a crucial role in their ability to overcome the mucus barrier (Dong et al. 2020).

Justin Hanes and the collaborators first presented the concept of mucus-penetrating particles, which were inspired by virus diffusion via mucous (Xu et al. 2013; Lai, Wang, and Hanes 2009). These particles, coated with low molecular weight PEG, imitate virus surface characteristics, thereby, decreasing interactions with mucus components and increasing penetration. PEG's hydrophilic and nearly neutrally charged surfaces allow for fast diffusion across the mucus layer (Xu et al. 2013; Lai, Wang, and Hanes 2009).

Furthermore, heavily PEGylated systems have been demonstrated to move through extremely viscous mucus samples, highlighting their potential for therapeutic applications. In addition, polymers such as poloxamer 407 have shown potential to enhance mucus penetration, with functionalized nanoparticles demonstrating increased permeability and cellular uptake when compared to unmodified ones (Lai, Wang, and Hanes 2009; Dong et al. 2020).

Alternative polymers for mucus-penetrating nanoparticles, in addition to PEG, include polysarcosine, poly(2-alkyl-2-oxazoline)s, and polyglycidols. These polymers have benefits such as biocompatibility and low immunogenicity, making them interesting for biomedical applications (Khutoryanskiy 2018; Ways et al. 2022).

Zwitterionic polymers, which include both anionic and cationic groups, have also shown potential for mucus penetration. These polymers have stealth-like properties, reducing protein adsorption and bacterial adhesion while increasing nanoparticle stability and dispersion in biological fluids (Ma et al. 2023).

Furthermore, the introduction of mucolytic enzymes in nanoparticulate systems has been investigated to improve particle diffusion across the mucous layer. Papain nanoparticles, for example, have been demonstrated to reduce mucus viscosity, allowing them to pass through the mucus layer more quickly. Similarly, bromelain-conjugated nanoparticles have a higher mucus-penetrating capacity than those without enzyme conjugation (Pereira De Sousa et al. 2015; Subramanian, Langer, and Traverso 2022).

Despite these advances, more research is needed to understand the synergistic effects of mixing polymeric particles with mucolytic agents, as well as the impact on local viscosity reduction and drug absorption. Continued investigation of innovative polymer-based techniques holds promise for breaking down the mucus barrier and enhancing the efficacy of drugs delivery systems (Subramanian, Langer, and Traverso 2022; Yan and Sha 2023).

4.6 BIOADHESIVE SYSTEMS APLICATION ON 3D PRINTING

3D printing has developed as an innovative technology in a variety of areas, including the pharmaceutical industry. In this context, 3D printing for bioadhesive drug delivery systems is a new, promising research area. The combination of the precision of 3D printing technology with the bioadhesive characteristics of the compounds used, producing devices that can adhere to the target biological surface and release medications in controlled ways over time.

One of the most impressive characteristics of these systems is their individualization, allowing the development of devices personalized to each patient's specifications. This technology offers the ability to develop extremely efficient and precise medicines that are customized to individual anatomy and physiology.

Furthermore, 3D printing permits multiple drugs to be incorporated into a single device, allowing for combination therapy to treat complex diseases. This versatility is especially important in the management of chronic diseases, where multiple treatment drugs may be required to control symptoms and improve the patient's quality of life.

Another important factor is the capacity to control drug release according to a predetermined frequency. This is accomplished by adjusting the device shape and the properties of the components utilized, allowing for the progressive release of the drug over time while avoiding potentially dangerous drugs concentration peaks.

Bioadhesive drug delivery systems developed by 3D printing have potential applications in a variety of medical areas. They can be used to treat dermatological conditions such as chronic wounds and burns, where device adherence to the skin is critical for successful drug delivery. Furthermore, these devices can be employed in difficult-to-reach areas of the organism, such as the gastrointestinal tract and ocular tissue, where adhesion is necessary for effective drug absorption.

Despite its many advantages, 3D printing of bioadhesive drug delivery devices presents significant challenges. To ensure the efficacy and safety of the manufactured devices, materials must be carefully selected, and printing conditions optimized. Furthermore, regulatory and production scaling challenges must be resolved before be commercialized.

To summarize, 3D printing of bioadhesive drug delivery devices is a promising research and development topic in modern medicine. With continued technological advancements and increased collaboration among researchers, physicians, and manufacturers this innovative approach has the potential to further revolutionize the field of drug therapy, providing more effective and personalized treatments for a wide range of medical conditions.

REFERENCES

Abrami, Michela, Alice Biasin, Fabiana Tescione, Domenico Tierno, Barbara Dapas, Annalucia Carbone, Gabriele Grassi, et al. 2024. "Mucus Structure, Viscoelastic Properties, and Composition in Chronic Respiratory Diseases." *International Journal of Molecular Sciences* 25 (3). https://doi.org/10.3390/ijms25031933.

Acartürk, Füsun. 2009. "Mucoadhesive Vaginal Drug Delivery Systems." *Recent Patents on Drug Delivery & Formulation* 3 (3): 193–205.

Ahmed, Sadek, Maha M. Amin, and Sinar Sayed. 2023. "Ocular Drug Delivery: A Comprehensive Review." *AAPS PharmSciTech* 24 (2). https://doi.org/10.1208/s12249-023-02516-9.

Amorós-Galicia, Lola, Anna Nardi-Ricart, Clara Verdugo-González, Carmen Martina Arroyo-García, Encarna García-Montoya, Pilar Pérez-Lozano, Josep Mª Suñé-Negre, and Marc Suñé-Pou. 2022. "Development of a Standardized Method for Measuring Bioadhesion and Mucoadhesion That Is Applicable to Various Pharmaceutical Dosage Forms." *Pharmaceutics* 14 (10). https://doi.org/10.3390/pharmaceutics14101995.

Anand, Utkarshini, Tiam Feridooni, and Remigius U. Agu. 2012. "Novel Mucoadhesive Polymers for Nasal Drug Delivery." In *Recent Advances in Novel Drug Carrier Systems*. InTech.

Andrade, Ana Ochoa, María Emma Parente, and Gastón Ares. 2014. "Screening of Mucoadhesive Vaginal Gel Formulations." *Brazilian Journal of Pharmaceutical Sciences* 50 (4): 931–42. https://doi.org/10.1590/S1984-82502014000400029.

Araújo, Mónica, Ana Camila Marques, José Manuel Sousa Lobo, and Maria Helena Amaral. 2022. "Semisolid Formulations Based on Solid-in-Oil-in-Water Systems Containing Proteins." *Brazilian Journal of Pharmaceutical Sciences* 58: 1–8. https://doi.org/10.1590/s2175-97902022e191093.

Arshad, Rabia, Muhammad Salman Arshad, Tanveer A. Tabish, Syed Nisar Hussain Shah, Saira Afzal, and Gul Shahnaz. 2022. "Amidated Pluronic Decorated Muco-Penetrating Self-Nano Emulsifying Drug Delivery System (SNEDDS) for Improved Anti-Salmonella Typhi Potential." *Pharmaceutics* 14 (11). https://doi.org/10.3390/pharmac eutics14112433.

Bansil, Rama, and Bradley S. Turner. 2018. "The Biology of Mucus: Composition, Synthesis and Organization." *Advanced Drug Delivery Reviews* 124: 3–15. https://doi.org/10.1016 /j.addr.2017.09.023.

Baranowski, Przemysław, Bozena Karolewicz, Maciej Gajda, and Janusz Pluta. 2014. "Ophthalmic Drug Dosage Forms: Characterisation and Research Methods." *The Scientific World Journal* 2014. https://doi.org/10.1155/2014/861904.

Barmpatsalou, Vicky. 2023. *Understanding the Gastrointestinal Mucus and Its Impact on Drug Absorption.* http://urn.kb.se/resolve?urn=urn:nbn:se:uu:diva-495168.

Basit, Abdul W., and Sarah J. Trenfield. 2022. "3D Printing of Pharmaceuticals and the Role of Pharmacy." *Pharmaceutical Journal* 308 (7959): 1–32. https://doi.org/10.1211/PJ .2022.1.135581.

Bayer, Ilker S. 2022. "Recent Advances in Mucoadhesive Interface Materials, Mucoadhesion Characterization, and Technologies." *Advanced Materials Interfaces* 9 (18). https://doi .org/10.1002/admi.202200211.

Bernkop-Schnürch, Andreas, Veronika Schwarz, and Sonja Steininger. 1999. "Polymers with Thiol Groups: A New Generation of Mucoadhesive Polymers?" *Pharmaceutical Research* 16.

Bitter, Christoph, Katja Suter-Zimmermann, and Christian Surber. 2011. "Nasal Drug Delivery in Humans." In *Topical Applications and the Mucosa.* Karger.

Boddupalli, Bindu M., Zulkar N.K. Mohammed, Ravinder Nath A., and David Banji. 2010. "Mucoadhesive Drug Delivery System: An Overview." *Journal of Advanced Pharmaceutical Technology and Research* 1 (4): 381–87. https://doi.org/10.4103/0110 -5558.76436.

Boegh, Marie, and Hanne Mørck Nielsen. 2015. "Mucus as a Barrier to Drug Delivery - Understanding and Mimicking the Barrier Properties." *Basic and Clinical Pharmacology and Toxicology* 116 (3): 179–86. https://doi.org/10.1111/bcpt.12342.

Bourlais, Chrystèle Le, Liliane Acar, Hosein Zia, Pierre A. Sado, Thomas Needham, and Roger Leverge. 1998. "Ophthalmic Drug Delivery Systems - Recent Advances." *Progress in Retinal and Eye Research* 17 (1): 33–58. https://doi.org/10.1016/S1350 -9462(97)00002-5.

Bu, Yazhong, and Abhay Pandit. 2022. "Cohesion Mechanisms for Bioadhesives." *Bioactive Materials* 13 (October 2021): 105–18. https://doi.org/10.1016/j.bioactmat.2021.11.008.

Burhan, Ayah Mohammad, Butsabarat Klahan, Wayne Cummins, Vanessa Andrés-Guerrero, Mark E. Byrne, Niall J. O'reilly, Anuj Chauhan, Laurence Fitzhenry, and Helen Hughes. 2021. "Posterior Segment Ophthalmic Drug Delivery: Role of Muco-Adhesion with a Special Focus on Chitosan." *Pharmaceutics* 13 (10). https://doi.org/10.3390/pharmac eutics13101685.

Carvalho, Flávia Chiva, Marcos Luciano Bruschi, Raul Cesar Evangelista, and Maria Palmira Daflon Gremião. 2010. "Mucoadhesive Drug Delivery Systems." *Brazilian Journal of Pharmaceutical Sciences* 46.

Castro-Balado, Ana, Cristina Mondelo-García, Irene Zarra-Ferro, and Anxo Fernández-Ferreiro. 2020. "New Ophthalmic Drug Delivery Systems." *Farmacia Hospitalaria* 44 (4): 149–57. https://doi.org/10.7399/fh.11388.

Cencer, Morgan, Yuan Liu, Audra Winter, Meridith Murley, Hao Meng, and Bruce P. Lee. 2014. "Effect of PH on the Rate of Curing and Bioadhesive Properties of Dopamine Functionalized Poly(Ethylene Glycol) Hydrogels." *Biomacromolecules* 15 (8): 2861–69. https://doi.org/10.1021/bm500701u.

Chan, Alistair K.C., Nehil Ranjitham Gopalakrishnan, Yannick Leandre Traore, and Emmanuel A. Ho. 2024. "Formulating Biopharmaceuticals Using Three-Dimensional Printing." *Journal of Pharmacy and Pharmaceutical Sciences* 27 (March): 1–15. https://doi.org/10.3389/jpps.2024.12797.

Charitakis, Alexandros, Sulaf Assi, Sakib Yousaf, and Iftikhar Khan. 2022. "Overcoming Skin Damage from Pollution via Novel Skincare Strategies." *Current Pharmaceutical Design* 28 (15): 1250–57. https://doi.org/10.2174/1381612828666220331124025.

Chaturvedi, Mayank, Manish Kumar, and Kamla Pathak. 2011. "A Review on Mucoadhesive Polymer Used in Nasal Drug Delivery System." *Journal of Advanced Pharmaceutical Technology and Research* 2 (4): 215–22. https://doi.org/10.4103/2231-4040.90876.

Cheung, Randy Chi Fai, Tzi Bun Ng, Jack Ho Wong, and Wai Yee Chan. 2015. *Chitosan: An Update on Potential Biomedical and Pharmaceutical Applications. Marine Drugs.* Vol. 13. https://doi.org/10.3390/md13085156.

Chinna Reddy, P., K. S.C. Chaitanya, and Y. Madhusudan Rao. 2011. "A Review on Bioadhesive Buccal Drug Delivery Systems: Current Status of Formulation and Evaluation Methods." *DARU, Journal of Pharmaceutical Sciences* 19 (6): 385–403.

Chonkar, Ankita, Usha Nayak, and N. Udupa. 2015. "Smart Polymers in Nasal Drug Delivery." *Indian Journal of Pharmaceutical Sciences* 77 (4): 367–75. https://doi.org/10.4103/0250-474X.164770.

Cortés, Hernán, Héctor Hernández-Parra, Sergio A. Bernal-Chávez, María L. Del Prado-Audelo, Isaac H. Caballero-Florán, Fabiola V. Borbolla-Jiménez, Maykel González-Torres, Jonathan J. Magaña, and Gerardo Leyva-Gómez. 2021. "Non-Ionic Surfactants for Stabilization of Polymeric Nanoparticles for Biomedical Uses." *Materials* 14 (12). https://doi.org/10.3390/ma14123197.

Curnutt, Austin, Kaylee Smith, Emily Darrow, and Keisha B. Walters. 2020. "Chemical and Microstructural Characterization of PH and [Ca2+] Dependent Sol-Gel Transitions in Mucin Biopolymer." *Scientific Reports* 10 (1): 21–23. https://doi.org/10.1038/s41598-020-65392-4.

Dartt, D. A. 1992. "Physiology of Tear Production." In *The Dry Eye*, 65–99. https://doi.org/10.1007/978-3-642-58130-4_4.

Das, Sabya Sachi, Priyanshu Bharadwaj, Muhammad Bilal, Mahmood Barani, Abbas Rahdar, Pablo Taboada, Simona Bungau, and George Z. Kyzas. 2020. "Stimuli-Responsive Polymeric Nanocarriers for Drug Delivery, Imaging, and Theragnosis." *Polymers* 12 (6). https://doi.org/10.3390/polym12061397.

Davis, Jordan D., and Tomasz P. Wypych. 2021. "Cellular and Functional Heterogeneity of the Airway Epithelium." *Mucosal Immunology* 14 (5): 978–90. https://doi.org/10.1038/s41385-020-00370-7.

Deng, Tuo, Dongxiu Gao, Xuemei Song, Zhipeng Zhou, Lixiao Zhou, Maixian Tao, Zexiu Jiang, et al. 2023. "A Natural Biological Adhesive from Snail Mucus for Wound Repair." *Nature Communications* 14 (1): 1–18. https://doi.org/10.1038/s41467-023-35907-4.

Desai, Nimeet, Dhwani Rana, Sagar Salave, Raghav Gupta, Pranav Patel, Bharathi Karunakaran, Amit Sharma, Jyotsnendu Giri, Derajram Benival, and Nagavendra Kommineni. 2023. "Chitosan: A Potential Biopolymer in Drug Delivery and Biomedical Applications." *Pharmaceutics* 15 (4). https://doi.org/10.3390/pharmaceutics15041313.

Dey, Aishee, Bhattacharya, and Sudarsan Neogi. 2021. "Bioadhesives in Biomedical Applications: A Critical Review." In *Progress in Adhesion and Adhesives*. John Wiley & Sons.

Dong, Wujun, Jun Ye, Junzhuo Zhou, Weijue Wang, Hongliang Wang, Xu Zheng, Yanfang Yang, Xuejun Xia, and Yuling Liu. 2020. "Comparative Study of Mucoadhesive and Mucus-Penetrative Nanoparticles Based on Phospholipid Complex to Overcome the Mucus Barrier for Inhaled Delivery of Baicalein." *Acta Pharmaceutica Sinica B* 10 (8): 1576–85. https://doi.org/10.1016/j.apsb.2019.10.002.

Eid, Ahmad M., Nagib A. Elmarzugi, and Nidal A. Jaradat. 2019. "Influence of Sonication and in Vitro Evaluation of Nifedipine Self-Nanoemulsifying Drug Delivery System." *Brazilian Journal of Pharmaceutical Sciences* 55: 1–8. https://doi.org/10.1590/s2175 -97902019000217497.

Ezike, Tobechukwu Christian, Ugochukwu Solomon Okpala, Ufedo Lovet Onoja, Chinenye Princess Nwike, Emmanuel Chimeh Ezeako, Osinachi Juliet Okpara, Charles Chinkwere Okoroafor, et al. 2023. "Advances in Drug Delivery Systems, Challenges and Future Directions." *Heliyon* 9 (6). https://doi.org/10.1016/j.heliyon.2023.e17488.

Federer, Christoph, Markus Kurpiers, and Andreas Bernkop-Schnürch. 2021. "Thiolated Chitosans: A Multi-Talented Class of Polymers for Various Applications." *Biomacromolecules* 22 (1): 24–56. https://doi.org/10.1021/acs.biomac.0c00663.

Fortuna, Ana, Katharina Schindowski, and Fabio Sonvico. 2022. "Intranasal Drug Delivery: Challenges and Opportunities." *Frontiers in Pharmacology* 13 (March): 10–12. https:// doi.org/10.3389/fphar.2022.868986.

Froelich, Anna, Emilia Jakubowska, Barbara Jadach, Piotr Gadziński, and Tomasz Osmałek. 2023. "Natural Gums in Drug-Loaded Micro- and Nanogels." *Pharmaceutics* 15 (3). https://doi.org/10.3390/pharmaceutics15030759.

Gavrovic-Jankulovic, Marija, and Radivoje Prodanovic. 2011. "Drug Delivery: Plant Lectins as Bioadhesive Drug Delivery Systems." *Journal of Biomaterials and Nanobiotechnology* 2 (5): 614–21. https://doi.org/10.4236/jbnb.2011.225073.

Gilhotra, Ritu M., Mohd Ikram, Sunny Srivastava, and Neeraj Gilhotra. 2014. "A Clinical Perspective on Mucoadhesive Buccal Drug Delivery Systems." *Journal of Biomedical Research* 28 (2): 81–97. https://doi.org/10.7555/JBR.27.20120136.

Grondin, Jensine A., Yun Han Kwon, Parsa Mehraban Far, Sabah Haq, and Waliul I. Khan. 2020. "Mucins in Intestinal Mucosal Defense and Inflammation: Learning From Clinical and Experimental Studies." *Frontiers in Immunology* 11 (September): 1–19. https://doi.org/10.3389/fimmu.2020.02054.

Grosso, Chelsey A. Del, Chuan Leng, Kexin Zhang, Hsiang Chieh Hung, Shaoyi Jiang, Zhan Chen, and Jonathan J. Wilker. 2020. "Surface Hydration for Antifouling and Bio-Adhesion." *Chemical Science* 11 (38): 10367–77. https://doi.org/10.1039/d0sc03690k.

Hagesaether, Ellen, and Sverre Arne Sande. 2007. "In Vitro Measurements of Mucoadhesive Properties of Six Types of Pectin." *Drug Development and Industrial Pharmacy* 33 (4): 417–25. https://doi.org/10.1080/03639040600920630.

Heikal, Eman J., Taha M. Hammady, and Shadeed Gad. 2016. "Bioadhesive Drug Delivery Systems : A Review." *Records of Pharmaceutical and Biomedical Sciences*.

Herath, Madushani, Suzanne Hosie, Joel C. Bornstein, Ashley E. Franks, and Elisa L. Hill-Yardin. 2020. "The Role of the Gastrointestinal Mucus System in Intestinal Homeostasis: Implications for Neurological Disorders." *Frontiers in Cellular and Infection Microbiology* 10 (May). https://doi.org/10.3389/fcimb.2020.00248.

Hill, David B., Paula A. Vasquez, John Mellnik, Scott A. McKinley, Aaron Vose, Frank Mu, Ashley G. Henderson, et al. 2014. "A Biophysical Basis for Mucus Solids Concentration as a Candidate Biomarker for Airways Disease." *PLoS ONE* 9 (2): 1–11. https://doi.org /10.1371/journal.pone.0087681.

Homayun, Bahman, Xueting Lin, and Hyo Jick Choi. 2019. "Challenges and Recent Progress in Oral Drug Delivery Systems for Biopharmaceuticals." *Pharmaceutics* 11 (3). https:// doi.org/10.3390/pharmaceutics11030129.

Hoti, Gjylije, Fabrizio Caldera, Claudio Cecone, Alberto Rubin Pedrazzo, Anastasia Anceschi, Silvia Lucia Appleton, Yousef Khazaei Monfared, and Francesco Trotta. 2021. "Effect of the Cross-Linking Density on the Swelling and Rheological Behavior of Ester-Bridged β-Cyclodextrin Nanosponges." *Materials* 14 (3): 1–20. https://doi.org /10.3390/ma14030478.

Huang, Xiaowei, Yankun Zheng, Jinfa Ming, Xin Ning, and Shumeng Bai. 2024. "Natural Polymer-Based Bioadhesives as Hemostatic Platforms for Wound Healing." *International Journal of Biological Macromolecules* 256 (June 2023). https://doi.org/10.1016/j.ijbiomac.2023.128275.

Inchaurraga, Laura, Nekane Martín-Arbella, Virginia Zabaleta, Gemma Quincoces, Ivan Peñuelas, and Juan M. Irache. 2015. "In Vivo Study of the Mucus-Permeating Properties of PEG-Coated Nanoparticles Following Oral Administration." *European Journal of Pharmaceutics and Biopharmaceutics* 97: 280–89. https://doi.org/10.1016/j.ejpb.2014.12.021.

Jackson, Kristin, and Kenneth J. Ii Miller. 2008. Transdermal systems containing multilayer adhesive matrices to modify drug delivery, issued 2008.

Jelkmann, Max, Christina Leichner, Sergey Zaichik, Flavia Laffleur, and Andreas Bernkop-Schnürch. 2020. "A Gellan Gum Derivative as In-Situ Gelling Cationic Polymer for Nasal Drug Delivery." *International Journal of Biological Macromolecules* 158: 1037–46. https://doi.org/10.1016/j.ijbiomac.2020.04.114.

Jeong, Woo Yeup, Mina Kwon, Hye Eun Choi, and Ki Su Kim. 2021. "Recent Advances in Transdermal Drug Delivery Systems: A Review." *Biomaterials Research* 25.

Ji, Xiaolong, Mingsong Yin, Hui Nie, and Yanqi Liu. 2020. "A Review of Isolation, Chemical Properties, and Bioactivities of Polysaccharides from Bletilla Striata." *BioMed Research International* 2020. https://doi.org/10.1155/2020/5391379.

Johansson, Malin E.V., Daniel Ambort, Thaher Pelaseyed, André Schütte, Jenny K. Gustafsson, Anna Ermund, Durai B. Subramani, et al. 2011. "Composition and Functional Role of the Mucus Layers in the Intestine." *Cellular and Molecular Life Sciences* 68 (22): 3635–41. https://doi.org/10.1007/s00018-011-0822-3.

Julião, Erielma Lomba Dias, Juliana Santos de Jesus Azevedo, Fábio Luís Menezes de Sousa, Alena Ribeiro Alves Peixoto Medrado, Juliana Borges de Lima Dantas, and Júlia Dos Santos Vianna Néri. 2022. "Evaluation of Topical Administration of Mucoadhesive Gel Containing Triamcinolone and Extracts of Aloe Vera and Propolis for Surgical Wound Tissue Repair in the Tongue of Rats." *Revista Brasileira de Plantas Medicinais* 24 (1): 29–37.

Kali, Gergely, Andrea Fürst, Nuri Ari Efiana, Aida Dizdarević, and Andreas Bernkop-Schnürch. 2023. "Intraoral Drug Delivery: Highly Thiolated κ-Carrageenan as Mucoadhesive Excipient." *Pharmaceutics* 15 (7). https://doi.org/10.3390/pharmaceutics15071993.

Kaur, Loveleen, and Inderbir Singh. 2020. "Chitosan-Catechol Conjugates–A Novel Class of Bioadhesive Polymers." In *Progress in Adhesion and Adhesives*. Wiley.

Ke, Xiang, Zhiyun Dong, Shuxian Tang, Wenlin Chu, Xiaoran Zheng, Li Zhen, Xingyu Chen, Chunmei Ding, Jun Luo, and Jianshu Li. 2020. "A Natural Polymer Based Bioadhesive with Self-Healing Behavior and Improved Antibacterial Properties." *Biomaterials Science* 8 (15): 4346–57. https://doi.org/10.1039/d0bm00624f.

Kedir, Welela Meka, Gamachu Fikadu Abdi, Meta Mamo Goro, and Leta Deressa Tolesa. 2022. "Pharmaceutical and Drug Delivery Applications of Chitosan Biopolymer and Its Modified Nanocomposite: A Review." *Heliyon* 8 (8). https://doi.org/10.1016/j.heliyon.2022.e10196.

Keller, Lea Adriana, Olivia Merkel, and Andreas Popp. 2022. "Intranasal Drug Delivery: Opportunities and Toxicologic Challenges during Drug Development." *Drug Delivery and Translational Research* 12 (4): 735–57. https://doi.org/10.1007/s13346-020-00891-5.

Khadem, Elham, Mahshid Kharaziha, Hamid Reza Bakhsheshi-Rad, Oisik Das, and Filippo Berto. 2022. *Cutting-Edge Progress in Stimuli-Responsive Bioadhesives: From Synthesis to Clinical Applications. Polymers.* Vol. 14. https://doi.org/10.3390/polym14091709.

Khutoryanskiy, Vitaliy V. 2018. "Beyond PEGylation: Alternative Surface-Modification of Nanoparticles with Mucus-Inert Biomaterials." *Advanced Drug Delivery Reviews* 124: 140–49. https://doi.org/10.1016/j.addr.2017.07.015.

Klemetsrud, Therese, Helene Jonassen, Marianne Hiorth, Anna Lena Kjøniksen, and Gro Smistad. 2013. "Studies on Pectin-Coated Liposomes and Their Interaction with Mucin." *Colloids and Surfaces B: Biointerfaces* 103: 158–65. https://doi.org/10.1016/j.colsurfb.2012.10.012.

Klitgaard, Mette, Jette Jacobsen, Maja Nørgaard Kristensen, Ragna Berthelsen, and Anette Müllertz. 2024. "Characterizing Interregional Differences in the Rheological Properties and Composition of Rat Small Intestinal Mucus." *Drug Delivery and Translational Research*, no. 0123456789. https://doi.org/10.1007/s13346-024-01574-1.

Knowles, Michael R., and Richard C. Boucher. 2002. "Mucus Clearance as a Primary Innate Defense Mechanism for Mammalian Airways." *Journal of Clinical Investigation* 109 (5): 571–77. https://doi.org/10.1172/JCI0215217.

Koutsoviti, Melitini, Angeliki Siamidi, Panagoula Pavlou, and Marilena Vlachou. 2021. "Recent Advances in the Excipients Used for Modified Ocular Drug Delivery." *Materials* 14 (15). https://doi.org/10.3390/ma14154290.

Kumar, Krishan, Neha Dhawan, Harshita Sharma, Shubha Vaidya, and Bhuvaneshwar Vaidya. 2014. "Bioadhesive Polymers: Novel Tool for Drug Delivery." *Artificial Cells, Nanomedicine and Biotechnology* 42 (4): 274–83. https://doi.org/10.3109/21691401.2013.815194.

Kumar, Lalit, Shivani Verma, Bhuvaneshwar Vaidya, and Vivek Gupta. 2017. "Bioadhesive Polymers for Targeted Drug Delivery." In *Nanotechnology-Based Approaches for Targeting and Delivery of Drugs and Genes*. Academic Press.

Lai, Samuel K., Ying Ying Wang, and Justin Hanes. 2009. "Mucus-Penetrating Nanoparticles for Drug and Gene Delivery to Mucosal Tissues." *Advanced Drug Delivery Reviews* 61 (2): 158–71. https://doi.org/10.1016/j.addr.2008.11.002.

Lankalapalli, S., and V.R.M. Kolapalli. 2009. "Polyelectrolyte Complexes: A Review of Their Applicability in Drug Delivery Technology." *Indian Journal of Pharmaceutical Sciences* 71 (5): 481–87. https://doi.org/10.4103/0250-474X.58165.

Laurén, Patrick, Heli Paukkonen, Tiina Lipiäinen, Yujiao Dong, Timo Oksanen, Heikki Räikkönen, Henrik Ehlers, Päivi Laaksonen, Marjo Yliperttula, and Timo Laaksonen. 2018. "Pectin and Mucin Enhance the Bioadhesion of Drug Loaded Nanofibrillated Cellulose Films." *Pharmaceutical Research* 35 (7). https://doi.org/10.1007/s11095-018-2428-z.

Lavelle, E. C., G. Grant, U. Pfuller, and D. T. O'Hagan. 2004. "Immunological Implications of the Use of Plant Lectins for Drug and Vaccine Targeting to the Gastrointestinal Tract." *Journal of Drug Targeting* 12 (2): 89–95. https://doi.org/10.1080/10611860410001693733.

Lavelle, E. C., G. Grant, A. Pusztal, U. Pfüller, and D. T. O'Hagan. 2000. "Mucosal Immunogenicity of Plant Lectins in Mice." *Immunology* 99 (1): 30–37. https://doi.org/10.1046/j.1365-2567.2000.00932.x.

Lee, Seung Hun, Se Kyoo Jeong, and Sung Ku Ahn. 2006. "An Update of the Defensive Barrier Function of Skin." *Yonsei Medical Journal* 47 (3): 293–306. https://doi.org/10.3349/ymj.2006.47.3.293.

Lehr, Claus Michael. 2000. "Lectin-Mediated Drug Delivery: The Second Generation of Bioadhesives." *Journal of Controlled Release* 65 (1–2): 19–29. https://doi.org/10.1016/S0168-3659(99)00228-X.

Leyva-Gómez, Gerardo, Elizabeth Piñón-Segundo, Néstor Mendoza-Muñoz, María L. Zambrano-Zaragoza, Susana Mendoza-Elvira, and David Quintanar-Guerrero. 2018. "Approaches in Polymeric Nanoparticles for Vaginal Drug Delivery: A Review of the State of the Art." *International Journal of Molecular Sciences* 19 (6): 1–19. https://doi.org/10.3390/ijms19061549.

Li Hai, Julien P. Limenitakis, Tobias Fuhrer, Markus B. Geuking, Melissa A. Lawson, Madeleine Wyss, Sandrine Brugiroux, et al. 2015. "The Outer Mucus Layer Hosts a Distinct Intestinal Microbial Niche." *Nature Communications* 6 (May). https://doi.org/10.1038/ncomms9292.

Li Shiding, Liangbo Chen, and Yao Fu. 2023. "Nanotechnology-Based Ocular Drug Delivery Systems: Recent Advances and Future Prospects." *Journal of Nanobiotechnology* 21 (1): 1–39. https://doi.org/10.1186/s12951-023-01992-2.

Lima, Caroline S.A. de, Justine P.R.O. Varca, Victória M. Alves, Kamila M. Nogueira, Cassia P.C. Cruz, M. Isabel Rial-Hermida, Sławomir S. Kadłubowski, Gustavo H.C. Varca, and Ademar B. Lugão. 2022. "Mucoadhesive Polymers and Their Applications in Drug Delivery Systems for the Treatment of Bladder Cancer." *Gels* 8 (9): 1–25. https://doi.org/10.3390/gels8090587.

Lou, Jie, Hongli Duan, Qin Qin, Zhipeng Teng, Fengxu Gan, Xiaofang Zhou, and Xing Zhou. 2023. "Advances in Oral Drug Delivery Systems: Challenges and Opportunities." *Pharmaceutics* 15 (2). https://doi.org/10.3390/pharmaceutics15020484.

Lu, Xiaoyan. 2018. "Polyelectrolyte Complexes Based on Poly (Acrylic Acid): Mechanics and Applications," no. 2018: 1–170.

Ludwig, Annick. 2005. "The Use of Mucoadhesive Polymers in Ocular Drug Delivery." *Advanced Drug Delivery Reviews* 57 (11): 1595–639. https://doi.org/10.1016/j.addr.2005.07.005.

Ma, Yubin, Yiyang Guo, Shan Liu, Yu Hu, Cheng Yang, Gang Cheng, Changying Xue, Yi Y. Zuo, and Bingbing Sun. 2023. "PH-Mediated Mucus Penetration of Zwitterionic Polydopamine-Modified Silica Nanoparticles." *Nano Letters* 23 (16): 7552–60. https://doi.org/10.1021/acs.nanolett.3c02128.

Macierzanka, Adam, Alan R. Mackie, and Lukasz Krupa. 2019. "Permeability of the Small Intestinal Mucus for Physiologically Relevant Studies: Impact of Mucus Location and Ex Vivo Treatment." *Scientific Reports* 9 (1): 1–12. https://doi.org/10.1038/s41598-019-53933-5.

Mahajan, Nilesh, Md Ali Mujtaba, Ritesh Fule, Sonali Thakre, Md Sayeed Akhtar, Sirajudeen S. Alavudeen, Md Khalid Anwer, Mohammed F. Aldawsari, Danish Mahmood, and Md Sarfaraz Alam. 2024. "Self-Emulsifying Drug Delivery System for Enhanced Oral Delivery of Tenofovir: Formulation, Physicochemical Characterization, and Bioavailability Assessment." *ACS Omega*. https://doi.org/10.1021/acsomega.3c08565.

Maisel, Katharina, Mihika Reddy, Qingguo Xu, Sumon Chattopadhyay, Richard Cone, Laura M. Ensign, and Justin Hanes. 2016. "Nanoparticles Coated with High Molecular Weight PEG Penetrate Mucus and Provide Uniform Vaginal and Colorectal Distribution in Vivo." *Nanomedicine* 11 (11): 1337–43. https://doi.org/10.2217/nnm-2016-0047.

Martau, Gheorghe Adrian, Mihaela Mihai, and Dan Cristian Vodnar. 2019. "The Use of Chitosan, Alginate, and Pectin in the Biomedical and Food Sector-Biocompatibility, Bioadhesiveness, and Biodegradability." *Polymers* 11 (11). https://doi.org/10.3390/polym11111837.

Martini, Daniela, Donato Angelino, Chiara Cortelazzi, Ivana Zavaroni, Giorgio Bedogni, Marilena Musci, Carlo Pruneti, et al. 2018. "Claimed Effects, Outcome Variables and Methods of Measurement for Health Claims Proposed under European Community Regulation 1924/2006 in the Framework of Maintenance of Skin Function." *Nutrients* 10 (1). https://doi.org/10.3390/nu10010007.

Miyazaki, Kaori, Akira Sasaki, and Hiroshi Mizuuchi. 2023. "Advances in the Evaluation of Gastrointestinal Absorption Considering the Mucus Layer." *Pharmaceutics* 15 (12). https://doi.org/10.3390/pharmaceutics15122714.

Mohammadzadeh, Ramin, and Yousef Javadzadeh. 2018. "An Overview on Oral Drug Delivery via Nano-Based Formulations." *Pharmaceutical and Biomedical Research* 4 (1): 1–7. https://doi.org/10.18502/pbr.v4i1.139.

Mohammed, Abdul Aleem, Mohammed S. Algahtani, Mohammad Zaki Ahmad, Javed Ahmad, and Sabna Kotta. 2021. "3D Printing in Medicine: Technology Overview and Drug Delivery Applications." *Annals of 3D Printed Medicine* 4. https://doi.org/10.1016/j.stlm.2021.100037.

Mohapatra, Snehamayee, Rajat Kumar Kar, Prasanta Kumar Biswal, and Sabitri Bindhani. 2022. "Approaches of 3D Printing in Current Drug Delivery." *Sensors International* 3 (November 2021). https://doi.org/10.1016/j.sintl.2021.100146.

Müller, Christiane, Glen Perera, Verena König, and Andreas Bernkop-Schnürch. 2014. "Development and in Vivo Evaluation of Papain-Functionalized Nanoparticles." *European Journal of Pharmaceutics and Biopharmaceutics* 84 (1).

Nafee, Noha Adel, Fatma Ahmed Ismail, Nabila Ahmed Boraie, and Lobna Mohamed Mortada. 2004. "Mucoadhesive Delivery Systems. I. Evaluation of Mucoadhesive Polymers for Buccal Tablet Formulation." *Drug Development and Industrial Pharmacy* 30 (9): 985–93. https://doi.org/10.1081/DDC-200037245.

Neutsch, Lukas, Verena E. Plattner, Sonja Polster-Wildhofen, Agnes Zidar, Andreas Chott, Gerrit Borchard, Othmar Zechner, Franz Gabor, and Michael Wirth. 2011. "Lectin Mediated Biorecognition as a Novel Strategy for Targeted Delivery to Bladder Cancer." *Journal of Urology* 186 (4): 1481–88. https://doi.org/10.1016/j.juro.2011.05.040.

Nhàn, Nguyễn Thị Thanh, Daniel E. Maidana, and Kaori H. Yamada. 2023. "Ocular Delivery of Therapeutic Agents by Cell-Penetrating Peptides." *Cells* 12 (7): 1–18. https://doi.org/10.3390/cells12071071.

Oliveira, Rafaela Santos de, Nadine Lysyk Funk, Juliana dos Santos, Thayse Viana de Oliveira, Edilene Gadelha de Oliveira, Cesar Liberato Petzhold, Tania Maria Haas Costa, Edilson Valmir Benvenutti, Monique Deon, and Ruy Carlos Ruver Beck. 2023. "Bioadhesive 3D-Printed Skin Drug Delivery Polymeric Films: From the Drug Loading in Mesoporous Silica to the Manufacturing Process." *Pharmaceutics* 15 (1). https://doi.org/10.3390/pharmaceutics15010020.

Oprea, Madalina, and Stefan Ioan Voicu. 2020. "Recent Advances in Composites Based on Cellulose Derivatives for Biomedical Applications." *Carbohydrate Polymers* 247 (April). https://doi.org/10.1016/j.carbpol.2020.116683.

Osmałek, Tomasz, Anna Froelich, Barbara Jadach, Adam Tatarek, Piotr Gadzinski, Aleksandra Falana, Kinga Gralinska, et al. 2021. "Recent Advances in Polymer-Based Vaginal Drug Delivery Systems." *Pharmaceutics* 13 (6): 1–49. https://doi.org/10.3390/pharmaceutics13060884.

Packham, David E. 2011. "Theories of Fundamental Adhesion." In *Handbook of Adhesion Technology.* Springer-Verlag Berlin Heidelberg.

Palacio, Manuel L.B., and Bharat Bhushan. 2012. "Bioadhesion: A Review of Concepts and Applications." *Philosophical Transactions of the Royal Society A: Mathematical, Physical and Engineering Sciences* 370 (1967): 2321–47. https://doi.org/10.1098/rsta.2011.0483.

Pandey, Manisha, Hira Choudhury, Azila Abdul-Aziz, Subrat Kumar Bhattamisra, Bapi Gorain, Teng Carine, Tan Wee Toong, Ngiam Jing Yi, and Lim Win Yi. 2021. "Promising Drug Delivery Approaches to Treat Microbial Infections in the Vagina: A Recent Update." *Polymers* 23 (1): 1–65. https://doi.org/10.3390/polym13010026.

Paone, Paola, and Patrice D. Cani. 2020. "Mucus Barrier, Mucins and Gut Microbiota: The Expected Slimy Partners?" *Gut* 69 (12): 2232–43. https://doi.org/10.1136/gutjnl-2020-322260.

Park, H., and J. R. Robinson. 1987. "Mechanisms of Mucoadhesion of Poly(Acrylic Acid) Hydrogels." *Pharmaceutical Research* 4 (6): 457–64. https://doi.org/10.1023/a:1016467219657.

Peppas, Nicholas A., Brock Thomas, and James McGinity. 2011. "Molecular Aspects of Mucoadhesive Carrier Development for Drug Delivery and Improved Absorption." *Journal of Biomaterials Science, Polymer Edition* 23.

Pereira De Sousa, Irene, Beatrice Cattoz, Matthew D. Wilcox, Peter C. Griffiths, Robert Dalgliesh, Sarah Rogers, and Andreas Bernkop-Schnürch. 2015. "Nanoparticles Decorated with Proteolytic Enzymes, a Promising Strategy to Overcome the Mucus Barrier." *European Journal of Pharmaceutics and Biopharmaceutics* 97: 257–64. https://doi.org/10.1016/j.ejpb.2015.01.008.

Pham, Phuong, Susan Oliver, Edgar H.H. Wong, and Cyrille Boyer. 2021. "Effect of Hydrophilic Groups on the Bioactivity of Antimicrobial Polymers." *Polymer Chemistry* 12 (39): 5689–703. https://doi.org/10.1039/d1py01075a.

Porwal, Amit, and Kamla Pathak. 2023. "Bioadhesion: Fundamentals and Mechanisms." In *Adhesives in Biomedical Applications*. Wiley.

Prajapati, Shailesh T., and L. D. Patel. 2024. "Carrageenan: A Naturally Occurring Routinely Used Excipient," no. January 2007.

Puri, Vivek, Ameya Sharma, Pradeep Kumar, and Inderbir Singh. 2020. "Thiolation of Biopolymers for Developing Drug Delivery Systems with Enhanced Mechanical and Mucoadhesive Properties: A Review." *Polymers* 12 (8). https://doi.org/10.3390/polym12081803.

Račić, Anđelka, and Danina Krajišnik. 2023. "Biopolymers in Mucoadhesive Eye Drops for Treatment of Dry Eye and Allergic Conditions: Application and Perspectives." *Pharmaceutics* 15 (2). https://doi.org/10.3390/pharmaceutics15020470.

Ramadon, Delly, Maeliosa T.C. McCrudden, Aaron J. Courtenay, and Ryan F. Donnelly. 2022. "Enhancement Strategies for Transdermal Drug Delivery Systems: Current Trends and Applications." *Drug Delivery and Translational Research* 12 (4): 758–91. https://doi.org/10.1007/s13346-021-00909-6.

Roy, S., K. Pal, A. Anis, K. Pramanik, and B. Prabhakar. 2009. "Polymers in Mucoadhesive Drug-Delivery Systems: A Brief Note." *Designed Monomers and Polymers* 12 (6): 483–95. https://doi.org/10.1163/138577209X12478283327236.

Roy, Saroj Kumar, and Bala Prabhakar. 2010. "Bioadhesive Polymeric Platforms for Transmucosal Drug Delivery Systems - A Review." *Tropical Journal of Pharmaceutical Research* 9 (1): 91–104. https://doi.org/10.4314/tjpr.v9i1.52043.

Sabatino, Antonio Di, Giovanni Santacroce, Carlo Maria Rossi, Giacomo Broglio, and Marco Vincenzo Lenti. 2023. "Role of Mucosal Immunity and Epithelial–Vascular Barrier in Modulating Gut Homeostasis." *Internal and Emergency Medicine* 18 (6): 1635–46. https://doi.org/10.1007/s11739-023-03329-1.

Saha, Nibedita, Nabanita Saha, Tomas Sáha, Ebru Toksoy Öner, Urška Vrabič Brodnjak, Heinz Redl, Janek von Byern, and Petr Sáha. 2020. "Polymer Based Bioadhesive Biomaterials for Medical Application—a Perspective of Redefining Healthcare System Management." *Polymers* 12 (12): 1–19. https://doi.org/10.3390/polym12123015.

Sahi, Ajar Kumar, Pooja Verma, Pallawi, Kameshwarnath Singh, and Sanjeev Kumar Mahto. 2019. "Advancements and New Technologies in Drug Delivery System." In *Biomedical Engineering and Its Applications in Healthcare*. Springer.

Samaridou, Eleni, Konstantina Karidi, Irene Pereira de Sousa, Beatrice Cattoz, Peter Griffiths, Olga Kammona, Andreas Bernkop-Schnürch, and Costas Kiparissides. 2014. "Enzyme-Functionalized PLGA Nanoparticles with Enhanced Mucus Permeation Rate." *World Scientific*.

Sandri, G., S. Rossi, F. Ferrari, M. Bonferoni, and C. Caramella. 2015. "Mucoadhesive Polymers as Enabling Excipients for Oral Mucosal Drug Delivery." In *Oral Mucosal Drug Delivery and Therapy*. Springer.

Santos, A. F. S., M. D. C. Da Silva, T. H. Napoleão, P. M. G. Paiva, M. T. S. Correia, and L. C. B. B. Coelho. 2014. "Lectins: Function, Structure, Biological Properties and Potential Applications." *Current Topics in Peptide and Protein Research* 15: 41–62.

Sato, Hideyuki, Kohei Yamada, Masateru Miyake, and Satomi Onoue. 2023. "Recent Advancements in the Development of Nanocarriers for Mucosal Drug Delivery Systems to Control Oral Absorption." *Pharmaceutics* 15 (12): 1–20. https://doi.org/10.3390/pharmaceutics15122708.

Schmid, Roman, Meta Volcic, Stephan Fischer, Zhi Qu, Holger Barth, Amirali Popat, Frank Kirchhoff, and Mika Lindén. 2023. "Surface Functionalization Affects the Retention and Bio-Distribution of Orally Administered Mesoporous Silica Nanoparticles in a Colitis Mouse Model." *Scientific Reports* 13 (1): 1–17. https://doi.org/10.1038/s41598-023-47445-6.

Schubert, Mitchell L. 1979. "Regulation of Gastric Acid Secretion." *Annual Review Physiology*.

Seddiqi, Hadi, Erfan Oliaei, Hengameh Honarkar, Jianfeng Jin, Lester C. Geonzon, Rommel G. Bacabac, and Jenneke Klein-Nulend. 2021. *Cellulose and Its Derivatives: Towards Biomedical Applications. Cellulose.* Vol. 28. https://doi.org/10.1007/s10570-020-03674-w.

Shahid, Muhammad, Riaz Rajoka, Hafiza Mahreen Mehwish, Yiguang Wu, Liqing Zhao, Yasir Arfat, Kashif Majeed, and Shoaib Anwaar. 2020. "Chitin / Chitosan Derivatives and Their Interactions with Microorganisms : A Comprehensive Review and Future Perspectives." *Critical Reviews in Biotechnology* 8551. https://doi.org/10.1080/07388551.2020.1713719.

Shaikh, Rahamatullah, Thakur Raj Singh, Martin Garland, A. Woolfson, and Ryan Donnelly. 2011. "Mucoadhesive Drug Delivery Systems." *Journal of Pharmacy and Bioallied Sciences* 3 (1): 89–100. https://doi.org/10.4103/0975-7406.76478.

Sheng, Yong Hua, and Sumaira Z. Hasnain. 2022. "Mucus and Mucins : The Underappreciated Host Defence System." *Frontiers in Cellular and Infection Microbiology* 12.

Singh, Baljit, and Vikrant Sharma. 2014. "Correlation Study of Structural Parameters of Bioadhesive Polymers in Designing a Tunable Drug Delivery System." *Langmuir* 30 (28): 8580–91. https://doi.org/10.1021/la501529f.

Smart, John D. 2004. "Recent Developments in the Use of Bioadhesive Systems for Delivery of Drugs to the Oral Cavity." *Critical Reviews™ in Therapeutic Drug Carrier Systems* 21.

Smart, John D. 2005. "The Basics and Underlying Mechanisms of Mucoadhesion." *Advanced Drug Delivery Reviews* 57 (11): 1556–68. https://doi.org/10.1016/j.addr.2005.07.001.

Smoleński, Michał, Bożena Karolewicz, Anna M. Gołkowska, Karol P. Nartowski, and Katarzyna Małolepsza-Jarmołowska. 2021. "Emulsion-Based Multicompartment Vaginal Drug Carriers: From Nanoemulsions to Nanoemulgels." *International Journal of Molecular Sciences* 22 (12). https://doi.org/10.3390/ijms22126455.

Song, Chunyan, Zhenglong Chai, Si Chen, Hui Zhang, Xiaohong Zhang, and Yuping Zhou. 2023. "Intestinal Mucus Components and Secretion Mechanisms: What We Do and Do Not Know." *Experimental and Molecular Medicine* 55 (4): 681–91. https://doi.org/10.1038/s12276-023-00960-y.

Subramanian, Deepak A., Robert Langer, and Giovanni Traverso. 2022. "Mucus Interaction to Improve Gastrointestinal Retention and Pharmacokinetics of Orally Administered Nano-Drug Delivery Systems." *Journal of Nanobiotechnology* 20 (1): 1–23. https://doi.org/10.1186/s12951-022-01539-x.

Sudhakar, Yajaman, Ketousetuo Kuotsu, and A. K. Bandyopadhyay. 2006. "Buccal Bioadhesive Drug Delivery - A Promising Option for Orally Less Efficient Drugs." *Journal of Controlled Release* 114 (1): 15–40. https://doi.org/10.1016/j.jconrel.2006.04 .012.

Suharyani, Ine, Ahmed Fouad Abdelwahab Mohammed, Muchtaridi Muchtaridi, Nasrul Wathoni, and Marline Abdassah. 2021. "Evolution of Drug Delivery Systems for Recurrent Aphthous Stomatitis." *Drug Design, Development and Therapy* 15: 4071– 89. https://doi.org/10.2147/DDDT.S328371.

Tarabova, L., Z. Makova, E. Piesova, R. Szaboova, and Z. Faixova. 2016. "Intestinal Mucus Layer and Mucins." *Folia Veterinaria* 60 (1): 21–25. https://doi.org/10.1515/fv-2016 -0003.

Tewari, Akhilesh Kumar, Satish Chandra Upadhyay, Manish Kumar, Kamla Pathak, Deepak Kaushik, Ravinder Verma, Shailendra Bhatt, Ehab El Sayed Massoud, Md Habibur Rahman, and Simona Cavalu. 2022. "Insights on Development Aspects of Polymeric Nanocarriers: The Translation from Bench to Clinic." *Polymers* 14 (17). https://doi.org /10.3390/polym14173545.

Thacker, Minal, Ching-li Tseng, Chih-yen Chang, and Subhaini Jakfar. 2020. "Mucoadhesive Bletilla Striata Polysaccharide-Based Artificial Tears to Relieve Symptoms and Inflammation in Rabbit with Dry Eyes Syndrome." *Polymers* 12 (7): 1–17.

Thirawong, Nartaya, Ross A. Kennedy, and Pornsak Sriamornsak. 2008. "Viscometric Study of Pectin-Mucin Interaction and Its Mucoadhesive Bond Strength." *Carbohydrate Polymers* 71 (2): 170–79. https://doi.org/10.1016/j.carbpol.2007.05.026.

Ugoeze, Kenneth Chinedu. 2020. "Bioadhesive Polymers for Drug Delivery Applications." In *Bioadhesives in Drug Delivery*. Wiley.

Uma, K. 2023. "Bioadhesives for Clinical Applications – A Mini Review." *Materials Advances* 4 (9): 2062–69. https://doi.org/10.1039/d2ma00941b.

Umamaheshwari, R. B., Suman Ramteke, and Narendra Kumar Jain. 2004. "Anti-Helicobacter Pylori Effect of Mucoadhesive Nanoparticles Bearing Amoxicilin in Experimental Gerbils Model." *AAPS PharmSciTech* 5 (2). https://doi.org/10.1208/pt050232.

Vargason, Ava M., Aaron C. Anselmo, and Samir Mitragotri. 2021. "The Evolution of Commercial Drug Delivery Technologies." *Nature Biomedical Engineering* 5 (September).

Vigani, Barbara, Silvia Rossi, Giuseppina Sandri, Maria Cristina Bonferoni, and Carla M. Caramella. 2023. "Mucoadhesive Polymers in Substance-Based Medical Devices: Functional Ingredients or What Else?" *Frontiers in Drug Safety and Regulation* 3 (August): 1–13. https://doi.org/10.3389/fdsfr.2023.1227763.

Wallace, Louisa E., Mengying Liu, Frank J.M. van Kuppeveld, Erik de Vries, and Cornelis A.M. de Haan. 2021. "Respiratory Mucus as a Virus-Host Range Determinant." *Trends in Microbiology* 29 (11): 983–92. https://doi.org/10.1016/j.tim.2021.03.014.

Ways, Twana Mohammed M., Sergey K. Filippov, Samarendra Maji, Mathias Glassner, Michal Cegłowski, Richard Hoogenboom, Stephen King, Wing Man Lau, and Vitaliy V. Khutoryanskiy. 2022. "Mucus-Penetrating Nanoparticles Based on Chitosan Grafted with Various Non-Ionic Polymers: Synthesis, Structural Characterisation and Diffusion Studies." *Journal of Colloid and Interface Science* 626: 251–64. https://doi .org/10.1016/j.jcis.2022.06.126.

Ways, Twana Mohammed M., Wing Man Lau, and Vitaliy V. Khutoryanskiy. 2018. "Chitosan and Its Derivatives for Application in Mucoadhesive Drug Delivery Systems." *Polymers* 10 (3). https://doi.org/10.3390/polym10030267.

Williams, Olatunji W., Amir Sharafkhaneh, Victor Kim, Burton F. Dickey, and Christopher M. Evans. 2006. "Airway Mucus: From Production to Secretion." *American Journal of Respiratory Cell and Molecular Biology* 34 (5): 527–36. https://doi.org/10.1165/rcmb.2005-0436SF.

Woodley, John. 2012. "Bioadhesion: New Possibilities for Drug Administration?" *Clinical Pharmacokinetics* 40.

Wright, Leah, Timothy J. Barnes, Paul Joyce, and Clive A. Prestidge. 2022. "Optimisation of a High-Throughput Model for Mucus Permeation and Nanoparticle Discrimination Using Biosimilar Mucus." *Pharmaceutics* 14 (12). https://doi.org/10.3390/pharmaceutics14122659.

Wu, Sarah J., Jingjing Wu, Samuel J. Kaser, Heejung Roh, Ruth D. Shiferaw, Hyunwoo Yuk, and Xuanhe Zhao. 2024. "A 3D Printable Tissue Adhesive." *Nature Communications* 15 (1): 1–12. https://doi.org/10.1038/s41467-024-45147-9.

Xu, Qingguo, Nicholas J. Boylan, Shutian Cai, Bolong Miao, Himatkumar Patel, and Justin Hanes. 2013. "Scalable Method to Produce Biodegradable Nanoparticles That Rapidly Penetrate Human Mucus." *Journal of Controlled Release* 170 (2): 279–86. https://doi.org/10.1016/j.jconrel.2013.05.035.

Xu, Qingguo, Laura M. Ensign, Nicholas J. Boylan, Arne Schön, Xiaoqun Gong, Jeh Chang Yang, Nicholas W. Lamb, et al. 2015. "Impact of Surface Polyethylene Glycol (PEG) Density on Biodegradable Nanoparticle Transport in Mucus Ex Vivo and Distribution in Vivo." *ACS Nano* 9 (9): 9217–27. https://doi.org/10.1021/acsnano.5b03876.

Yan, Xin, and Xianyi Sha. 2023. "Nanoparticle-Mediated Strategies for Enhanced Drug Penetration and Retention in the Airway Mucosa." *Pharmaceutics* 15 (10). https://doi.org/10.3390/pharmaceutics15102457.

Yermak, Irina M., Viktoriya N. Davydova, and Aleksandra V. Volod'ko. 2022. "Mucoadhesive Marine Polysaccharides." *Marine Drugs* 20 (8). https://doi.org/10.3390/md20080522.

Younas, Farhan, Muhammad Zaman, Waqar Aman, Umer Farooq, Maria Abdul Ghafoor Raja, and Muhammad Wahab Amjad. 2023. "Thiolated Polymeric Hydrogels for Biomedical Applications: A Review." *Current Pharmaceutical Design* 29 (40): 3172–86. https://doi.org/10.2174/1381612829666230825100859.

Yu, Liu, Zewen Luo, Tian Chen, Yaqi Ouyang, Lingyun Xiao, Shu Liang, Zhangwen Peng, Yang Liu, and Yang Deng. 2022. "Bioadhesive Nanoparticles for Local Drug Delivery." *International Journal of Molecular Sciences* 23 (4). https://doi.org/10.3390/ijms23042370.

Yuan, Xiaozhi, Rajendran Amarnath Praphakar, Murugan A. Munusamy, Abdullah A. Alarfaj, Subbiah Suresh Kumar, and Mariappan Rajan. 2019. "Mucoadhesive Guargum Hydrogel Inter-Connected Chitosan-g-Polycaprolactone Micelles for Rifampicin Delivery." *Carbohydrate Polymers* 206 (September 2018): 1–10. https://doi.org/10.1016/j.carbpol.2018.10.098.

Zhu, Chen Yuan, Fei Long Li, Ye Wang Zhang, Rahul K. Gupta, Sanjay K.S. Patel, and Jung Kul Lee. 2022. "Recent Strategies for the Immobilization of Therapeutic Enzymes." *Polymers* 14 (7). https://doi.org/10.3390/polym14071409.

5 Biomaterials and Bioinks

5.1 3D BIOPRINTING

Bioprinting is the precise deposition of bioinks or biomaterial solutions to create 3D structures in layered formations. Bioprinting refers to operations involving living cells, in which the result is printed structures; in the absence of live cells, it is simply referred to as printing, with the structures acting as scaffolds (Li et al. 2020; Askari et al. 2021).

In recent years, bioprinting research has been emphasized and given significant attention. Due to this research, bioprinting has been found to be incredibly significant for various reasons. First, it permits the printing of 3D structures that can replicate the intricacy of human tissues. These structures can be utilized to repair damaged tissues or to build transplantable organs, reducing the demand for organ transplants. Second, by printing human tissues in a laboratory, researchers can investigate novel treatments and drugs in an accurate and ethical way, decreasing the demand for animal testing and accelerating the discovery of new treatments (Mendoza-Cerezo et al. 2023).

Furthermore, the ability to produce individual tissues and organs for each patient offers the possibility for personalized therapy. This means that professionals can create medicines that are personalized to the specific requirements of each patient, resulting in better therapeutic results. Bioprinting can also be used as a platform to support controlled and reproducible investigations into diseases and disorders. Researchers can create tissue models that replicate certain disease situations in order to better understand what causes them and discover novel treatments. Finally, 3D printed tissue models can be utilized to teach surgeons and other healthcare workers how to do complex surgical operations. This can increase the accuracy and safety of surgeries, reducing the risk to patients (Ma et al. 2018).

To summarize, bioprinting has the potential to transform medicine and biomedical research by providing new techniques to treat diseases, produce medications, and get greater comprehension of the human organism.

5.2 BIOINKS AND BIOMATERIALS

Biomaterials are materials or compounds that are utilized in biological systems such as cells, tissues, or organs. They can be natural or synthetic, and they have been developed to perform certain activities in biomedical contexts. Biomaterials can be utilized for a variety of purposes, including medical implants, medical devices, tissue engineering, medical diagnostics, regenerative medicine, and controlled drug delivery. The appropriate biomaterial is determined by what qualities are needed

DOI: 10.1201/9781003442363-5

for the individual application, such as biocompatibility, biodegradability, mechanical strength, and the ability to interact with cells and tissues (Kapusetti, More, and Choppadandi 2019).

During the 3D bioprinting, the formulations with biomaterial have additionally biological cells. These solutions (biomaterials and cells) used in the bioprinting process is known as "bioink" and it has an important part in the development of biological systems printed (Li et al. 2022).

In the context of tissue or organ bioprinting, bioink mostly refers to biological cells, which are essential for replication of the complex cellular architecture of realistic tissues. In contrast, scaffold bioprinting, which focuses on generating structural systems for tissue regeneration, often does not include cells in the formulation composition (Ramiah et al. 2020).

In addition to biological components, bioink formulations contain a wide variety of polymer compositions. These polymers act as scaffolding materials, providing the structural support and bioactive environment needed for cell adhesion, proliferation, and tissue formation. Depending on the application and desired qualities, these polymers can take many forms, such as individual hydrogels, polymers, or mixtures (N. Li, Guo, and Zhang 2021).

Polymers, which are long chains with a high-water content, have the advantage of producing a hydrated tissue-like environment that supports diverse cell processes required for tissue regeneration. These functions include crucial cellular activities such as adhesion, proliferation, and differentiation. Polymers can be divided into two types: natural and synthetic. Natural polymers have features that help cell function, making them ideal for biomedical applications. In contrast, synthetic polymers, while are often physiologically inert, have robust and long-lasting mechanical characteristics that improve the structural integrity of bioprinted constructions. This diversity of polymer types provides researchers with a wide range of materials for customizing bioinks to specific biomedical needs and applications (Wang 2019; Liu et al. 2022; Ramiah et al. 2020).

Furthermore, bioink formulations may contain other elements to improve performance and usefulness (Ji and Guvendiren 2017). These additions include bioceramic substances such as hydroxyapatite and tricalcium phosphate. These bioceramics have an important function in strengthening the polymer matrix, increasing mechanical strength, and facilitating cell–matrix interactions. Bioink formulations that incorporate these bioceramic components can imitate the natural environment of tissues, promoting tissue regeneration and functional integration after implantation (N. Li, Guo, and Zhang 2021; Fang et al. 2023; Ramiah et al. 2020).

5.3   COMPOSITION OF BIOINK

According to the definition, bioink is a complex formulation of cells that can be processed using controlled biofabrication technology. This formulation may also include physiologically active components and biomaterials, creating an environment for the complex structures needed in tissue engineering and regenerative medicine. The presence of a sufficient number of living cells in the bioink is critical because it provides for the precise organization of cells inside an appropriate spatial configuration during the printing process. However, the full application of functional organs requires further periods of incubation during which the cells proliferate, differentiate, and mature. As a result, cells are critical components of bioink, acting as the essential building blocks for tissue creation (Gopinathan and Noh 2018).

Furthermore, biomaterials are crucial components in the bioink formulation. They provide the essential support to maintain the spatial distribution of cells during the printing process (Ji and Guvendiren 2017; Freeman et al. 2022). Furthermore, biomaterials have an important role in sustaining cell viability during printing, increasing cellular proliferation and promoting differentiation after printing. Their intrinsic qualities, such as biocompatibility, biodegradability, and mechanical strength, help to ensure the overall success of the biofabrication process. Thus, the living cells and biomaterials within the bioink are critical for the successful construction of functional tissue structures with the necessary morphological and physiological properties (Ji and Guvendiren 2017; Freeman et al. 2022).

5.3.1 NATURAL-SOURCED MATERIALS

5.3.1.1 Alginate

Alginate, also known as alginic acid, is a water-soluble polysaccharide derived predominantly from brown seaweed and belongs to a significant family of natural polymers (Chen et al. 2023; Axpe and Oyen 2016). The monomers β-D-mannuronic acid (M) and α-L-guluronic acid (G) form homopolymeric blocks with consecutive G-residues (G-blocks), consecutive M-residues (M-blocks), or alternating M- and G-residues (MG-blocks). The different proportions of G and M blocks in alginate produce molecular weights ranging from 50 to 100,000 kDa (Axpe and Oyen 2016; Naghieh et al. 2018).

Alginate has been widely used in extrusion bioprinting due to its simplicity of printing, compatibility with ionic cross-linking, intrinsic water absorbency, and low cost. Alginate solutions used in bioprinting have demonstrated compatibility with a wide range of cell types generated from various tissues, including bone, muscle, cartilage, skin, neuron, and blood vessels, as well as functional organs including the heart, liver, kidney, and bladder (Gonzalez-Fernandez et al. 2021; Ahmadi Soufivand et al. 2023).

However, alginate has a significant disadvantage: low cell adherence. The absence of adhesion molecules within alginate or transmembrane glycoproteins significantly reduces the connection between cells and alginate limiting cell activity (Farshidfar, Iravani, and Varma 2023; Sahoo and Biswal 2021; Caliari and Burdick 2016). To solve this limitation, alginate's adhesion properties can be improved by incorporating other biomaterials with inherent cell attachment characteristics or by modifying it with specialized adhesion molecules sequences, which can form covalent bonds with alginate chains (Neves, Moroni, and Barrias 2020; Lee and Mooney 2012; Caliari and Burdick 2016; Farshidfar, Iravani, and Varma 2023).

5.3.1.2 Chitosan

Chitosan, a common natural polymer derived from crustacean shells and fungal cell walls, is produced through alkali deacetylation of chitin. The structure is a linear polysaccharide with randomly dispersed N-acetyl-D-glucosamine (acetylated units) and β-(1-4)-linked D-glucosamine (deacetylated units). Unlike chitin, chitosan dissolves quickly in dilute acidic environments below its pKa (pH = 6.5), but remains insoluble in common organic solvents (Sikorski, Gzyra-Jagieła, and Draczyński 2021; Roy et al. 2017; Nishimura et al. 1991).

Chitosan is well-known for its low cost and benefits, including non-toxicity, biodegradability, and antibacterial and antifungal qualities. It is used in a wide range of medical fields, from pharmaceuticals to wound dressings. It also has applications in bioprinting (Mora Boza et al. 2019; Lazaridou, Bikiaris, and Lamprou 2022; Mallakpour, Sirous, and Hussain 2021).

However, using traditional chitosan solutions for bioprinting cell-incorporated scaffolds presents difficulties due to the adverse acidic environment for cell viability. One strategy to overcoming this difficulty is to chemically change chitosan to make it water-soluble with a neutral pH after dissolution (Yusof et al. 2023; Roy et al. 2017; Chen et al. 2022).

Furthermore, the slow gel formation rate and fragile mechanical characteristics of chitosan present further challenges for bio-printing. These disadvantages can be addressed by combining chitosan solutions with other hydrogels such as gelatin, starch, collagen, pectin, and alginate, which improve polymerization rate and structural integrity (Mora Boza et al. 2019; Maiz-Fernández et al. 2022).

5.3.1.3 Agarose

Agarose, obtained from seaweed (red algae), is a naturally occurring water-soluble polymer that requires purifying processes. It has the peculiar property of self-cross-linking and de-cross-linking under temperature modulation. Agarose solutions gel rapidly around 26–30°C, making them ideal for printing. However, despite its applicability, some obstacles persist (Wenger et al. 2022; López-Marcial et al. 2018).

Because it is non-adhesive, agarose provides minimal support for cell development and dissolves over time. As a result, it is frequently used to generate cell aggregates or to promote the development of encapsulated cells. Collagen can be added to agarose solutions to improve its support for cellular activities such as protein and proteoglycan production, allowing living cells to be included (Salati et al. 2020; Mirdamadi et al. 2019).

Furthermore, because of its thermosensitivity, agarose is an important component in scaffold vascularization as a "sacrifice biomaterial." In this method, agarose fibers are printed in predetermined structures, then functional biomaterials and cells are inserted on them and cross-linked. The agarose fibers may be dissolved and removed easily using precise temperature control, leaving behind patterned channels for future use (Hauser et al. 2021; Mirdamadi et al. 2019; Kress et al. 2018; Kniebs et al. 2020).

5.3.1.4 Hyaluronic Acid

Hyaluronic acid is one of the most common glycosaminoglycans found in the extracellular matrix, with a large distribution across the human body's connective, epithelial, and neural tissues. Hyaluronic acid, known for its low inflammatory response and antigenic potential, is widely used in therapeutic applications as a dermal filler for wound healing and as synovial fluid in articular points due to its lubricating characteristics (Yasin et al. 2022).

Hyaluronic acid plays an important part in bioprinting, primarily as an auxiliary material used to modify the viscosity of other biomaterial solutions, due to its water solubility and high viscosity when dissolved. Its adaptable physical and biological characteristics make it an excellent candidate for setting cells into bioinks (Sekar et al. 2023; Hauptstein et al. 2020; Noh et al. 2019; Pereira et al. 2023).

However, hyaluronic acid's intrinsic limitations, such as its slow gelation rate, fragile mechanical properties, and rapid disintegration rate, demand alterations to make it more suitable for bioprinting applications. One technique is to alter hyaluronic acid with UV-curable methacrylate, which allows for photopolymerization while also enhancing cross-linking efficacy and mechanical stability for scaffold bioprinting (Li et al. 2023).

5.3.1.5 Collagen

Collagen, a protein found in abundance in the body, is composed of self-aggregating polypeptide chains linked together by hydrogen and covalent connections. It is a desirable material for tissue scaffolds due to its natural cell attachment receptors, which directly influence cell adhesion and other functions. Several varieties of collagens have been identified, some of which are better suited to bioprinting applications. Collagen types I, II, IV, and V are among the most used forms in tissue engineering, with collagen type I being particularly prevalent in scaffold bioprinting (Gibney, Patterson, and Ferraris 2021; Stepanovska et al. 2021).

While collagen scaffolds are compatible with a wide range of cell types, they face challenges due to their inherent low mechanical qualities. Collagen's suitability for scaffold bioprinting and tissue engineering has been improved through methods such as covalent bonding, irradiation cross-linking, and heat polymerization. In addition, collagen solutions have been combined with other materials such as alginate, gelatin, and hyaluronic acid to increase mechanical qualities in scaffold bioprinting (Guo et al. 2023; Osidak et al. 2020).

Collagen scaffolds are frequently used in the regeneration of hard tissues such as bone and cartilage, in addition to synthetic polymers such as polycaprolactone and poly(lactic-co-glycolic acid). In this method, synthetic polymers are printed first to provide mechanical support, followed by the deposition of collagen and cells within the scaffold's gaps to achieve biological functionalities (Dong and Lv 2016).

Although collagen is widely used in bioprinting, current studies are focused on enhancing its printability, gelation time, and cross-linking mechanisms. Strategies such as riboflavin photo cross-linking have been investigated to improve the printability of collagen inks, highlighting the significance of modulus in influencing printing quality. Furthermore, collagen can be integrated into other bioinks to increase bioactivity by offering diverse structures for cell adhesion and proliferation. In conclusion, collagen's versatility and bioactivity make it an important component in tissue engineering and bioprinting, with continuing research aimed at improving its properties for improved scaffold manufacturing and tissue regeneration (Osidak et al. 2020; Stepanovska et al. 2021; Liu et al. 2022; Nayak et al. 2023).

5.3.1.6 Gelatin

Gelatin, which is generated from collagen hydrolysis, has various advantages, including high biocompatibility, non-immunogenicity, cell affinity, and complete biodegradability in vivo. Gelatin, which has a comparable composition to collagen, is commonly used in tissue engineering applications. Like collagen, it is temperature sensitive and will cross-link at low temperatures. To improve its printability and stability for extrusion-based bioprinting, metal ions, glutaraldehyde, and other printable materials have been used (Wang et al. 2017; Lukin et al. 2022; Guo et al. 2023).

Chemical modification of gelatin has been investigated to create photo-cross-linkable gelatin hydrogels, such as gelatin methacrylate composite (GelMA) hydrogels. GelMA hydrogels have been successfully printed with UV light and used to encapsulate diverse cell types for the creation of tissue-engineered heart valves, cartilage, and vessel-like structures. The mechanical properties of modified gelatin can be controlled by changing factors such as gelatin concentration, UV light intensity, and exposure period (Bupphathong et al. 2022; Ghosh et al. 2023).

GelMA is the most widely used modified gelatin for bioprinting applications. Despite its promising qualities such as biocompatibility, mechanical properties, bioactivity, and biodegradability, the degree of functionalization is essential because it could affect the final result depending on the tissue type. For soft tissue engineering, low-methacrylate GelMA is suggested (Bupphathong et al. 2022; Applications 2022).

5.3.1.7 Fibrin

Fibrin, a fibrous protein that occurs naturally in the body during blood coagulation and is also a component of the natural extracellular matrix, has potential for a variety of 3D-biofabrication applications. Fibrinogen is a protein made up of two groups of three polypeptide chains (Aα, Bβ, and γ). Fibrinogen can be transformed into fibrin hydrogels by adding thrombin, a serine protease. Coagulation factor XIII crosslinks with the fibrin polymer's γ chains, creating a persistent network that is resistant to protease destruction (de Melo et al. 2020).

During bioprinting, fibrin can be easily created by immediately depositing a fibrinogen solution into a thrombin and factor XIII mixture. Fibrin-based scaffolds have inherent cell adhesion capacity, making them ideal for applications that require mixing cells with fibrinogen solutions to form cell-incorporated fibrin constructions that promote proliferation. However, their usefulness is limited by their low mechanical stability and quick deterioration rates (Gopinathan and Noh 2018; Cavallo et al. 2023).

Several approaches have been proposed to improve the mechanical characteristics of fibrin-based scaffolds. These include utilizing high quantities of fibrinogen or thrombin during fibrin production and adding additional biomaterials with greater mechanical stability. To slow down the rate of breakdown, protease inhibitors such as aprotinin can be added to fibrinogen solutions or culture medium. Optimization of printing factors such as temperature, calcium ion concentration, and cell density may help in degradation control (Rojas-Murillo et al. 2022; Sanz-Horta et al. 2023; Gopinathan and Noh 2018; de Melo et al. 2020).

Extrusion bioprinting of fibrin-based scaffolds is difficult due to the low viscosity of the fibrinogen solution. To improve viscosity, pre-mixed fibrinogen and thrombin solutions were used, which were normally produced at low temperatures to allow for mild gelation. Furthermore, fibrinogen has been mixed with various biomaterials during solution preparation and then cross-linked with associated cross-linkers to improve fibrin printability (de Melo et al. 2020).

5.3.2 Poly Caprolactone

Poly caprolactone (PCL) is an economically viable choice with exceptional bioink properties, such as hardness, biocompatibility, and degradability. In hard tissue engineering applications, it is mostly utilized for fused deposition modeling (FDM) and stereolithography (SLA). With a relatively low melting point of 60°C and acceptable rheological and viscoelastic qualities, PCL can be thermally treated for melt-based extrusion printing applications. It is considered as a non-toxic polymer with a notable stability of around 6 months and has a biological half-life of 3 years (Stafin, Śliwa, and Piątkowski 2023).

Scaffolds printed with selective laser sintering (SLS) and PCL have a porous structure with interconnectivity, a rough surface, and compactness equivalent to bone, which promotes bone repair and cell growth. However, PCL's prolonged biological half-life presents additional problems in applications across bone tissue engineering. Furthermore, its intrinsic hydrophobic properties contribute to low bioactivity, which slows cell development and tissue adherence (Gopinathan and Noh 2018).

PCL is a polyester that exhibits hydrolysis-induced biodegradation in physiological settings, making it ideal for tissue engineering applications such as drug administration and bone replacement. PCL's thermoplastic nature, high mechanical strength, and slow degradation profile make it ideal for 3D printing. However, due to their high melting temperature, PCL scaffolds usually require cell transplantation after construction, impregnation, or printing with another hydrogel bioink containing cells to generate a hybrid scaffold structure (Amni et al. 2021).

Combining PCL with other biocompatible polymers expands its possibilities in tissue engineering, including controlled bone regeneration membranes, surgical sutures, and drug-delivery capsules. Furthermore, combining PCL with polyethylene glycol (PEG) produces amphiphilic thermosensitive behavior, allowing for fast and reversible physical gelation under temperature control (Amni et al. 2021).

In addition, PCL's potential to form highly interconnected nano- and microfibers makes it excellent for building scaffolds using selective laser sintering (SLS) and digital light processing (DLP), which provide sufficient porosity for embedding cells, growth factors, drugs, and other bioactive substances (Amni et al. 2021).

5.3.3 POLY(ETHYLENE)-BASED POLYMERS

Poly(ethylene)-based polymers, particularly poly(ethylene glycol) (PEG) and poly(ethylene oxide) (PEO), are the most popular synthetic hydrogels in scaffold bioprinting for tissue engineering due to their adaptable attributes. These polymers are generated by polymerizing ethylene oxide and are classified as PEG or PEO based on their molecular weight. PEG and PEO have an incredible capacity to connect with water molecules, enhancing intraluminal water retention. Furthermore, their water solubility, metabolic inactivity, and biocompatibility help to minimize immunogenicity after implantation (Perez-Puyana et al. 2020).

PEG is a hydrophilic polymer generated through radical polymerization. Its superior biocompatibility has made it a popular material for drug delivery systems, tissue engineering scaffolds, and surface alterations. However, its non-biodegradability and low mechanical strength require adaptations for biomedical applications. Nonetheless, PEG breakdown can occur via hydrolytic and enzymatic mechanisms (Kohane and Langer 2008).

Hydrogels made from PEG and PEO have high permeability, which allows for nutrition and elimination of waste to support cell metabolism, making them ideal for cell encapsulation and delivery systems. However, their synthetic origin affects protein binding and cell adhesion. In order to solve this, modifications with peptides are popular, which improve cell adherence (Miller et al. 2010).

In scaffold bioprinting, PEG/PEO solutions are frequently modified to be photopolymerizable with acrylates or methacrylates, allowing for effective cross-linking by UV light and enhanced mechanical stability after extrusion. These hydrogels have uses in scaffold materials for cell encapsulation and vaccine delivery systems. Copolymerization with other synthetic polymers, such as polyvinyl alcohol (PVA), can be used to change the degradation properties (Perez-Puyana et al. 2020).

5.3.4 PLURONIC®

Pluronic® is a tri-block copolymer composed of poly(ethylene oxide) (PEO) and hydrophobic poly(propylene oxide) (PPO), with an triblock configuration (PEO–PPO–PEO). Its thermosensitive nature causes gelation when the PPO side chains become less soluble above a certain temperature limit, which typically ranges between 22 and 37°C, depending on polymer concentration.

Pluronic® displays surfactant qualities due to its amphiphilic features, which include the existence of both hydrophobic and hydrophilic segments. However, despite its benefits, Pluronic® has limitations. Its synthetic composition causes restricted cell adherence and disintegration, generating affects about its cytocompatibility, which could damage the cell membrane (Pitto-Barry and Barry 2014).

Despite these disadvantages, Pluronic® is useful as a "sacrificial" bioink, especially for constructing molds, channels, vessels, or vasculature in 3D bioprinting applications, or as a temporary support structure. Its high viscosity and great printability make it attractive for bioprinting structures with accurate shape fidelity, balancing its disadvantages (Pitto-Barry and Barry 2014).

5.3.5 Acrylonitrile Butadiene Styrene

Acrylonitrile butadiene styrene (ABS) emerges as a petrochemical triblock copolymer, making it one of the first plastics used in 3D printing. Unlike brittle polyester materials, ABS has impressive strength and flexibility, making it a popular alternative. ABS is remarkably resilient across a wide temperature range, from −20°C to 80°C, and has a melting point of 105°C, making it ideal for applications in FDM and SLA systems (Merazzo et al. 2023).

ABS is a petrochemical-derived triblock copolymer that belongs to the styrene terpolymer chemical family. It is made up of three different monomers, each of which has its own set of characteristics. Acrylonitrile improves heat resilience, butadiene increases impact strength, and styrene adds rigidity. These properties make ABS essential in a variety of technologies, including fused deposition modeling (FDM) and selective laser sintering (SLS) printing. Furthermore, ABS has applications in cartilage engineering (Merazzo et al. 2023).

However, its non-biodegradable nature, limited cell immigration, and mechanical properties, similar to polylactic acid (PLA), limit its application.

5.3.6 Polylactic Acid

Polylactic acid (PLA) is a hydrolytically degradable aliphatic polyester with biocompatibility, degradability, and printing properties, making it an effective polymeric bioink. PLA is the principal polymer used in the FDM technique for producing filaments that are used in muscles and bones tissue engineering, particularly for ligament substitutes and nonbiodegradable fibers (Castañeda-Rodríguez et al. 2023).

However, the degrading process of PLA produces acidic contaminants, which affects its long-term biocompatibility by causing tissue inflammation and cell death. Furthermore, PLA's inherent fragility, it is not as strong as bone, limits its usefulness. This problem can be solved by integrating low-cost ceramic materials such as calcium phosphate, resulting in scaffolds with improved bone strength and lower acid production (Chen et al. 2021).

5.3.7 Polycarbonate

Polycarbonate (PC) emerges as a biomaterial known for its great strength, which can sustain physical deformation up to over 150°C. However, PC's vulnerability to water absorption from the atmosphere limits its performance and printing durability (Lyu and Untereker 2009; Chen et al. 2023).

In recent applications, PC has found utility as a scaffold in medical contexts, due to its variable porosity ranging from 1% to 30% and excellent mechanical properties.

However, it is critical to remember that as the scaffold's porosity increases, these excellent mechanical performances may deteriorate (Chen et al. 2023).

5.3.8 POLYPROPYLENE

Polypropylene (PP) is a crystalline thermoplastic polymer made from propene monomer with a melting point of 165°C. With a density of 0.908 g/cm^3, PP is an excellent choice for applications where weight reduction is the main objective (Mattos et al. 2014; Shenoy and Patil 2010).

Additionally, PP is renowned for its resistance to abrasion and ability to absorb shocks, as well as its important hardness ranging from 1.2 to 1.6 GPa and strength at break ranging from 20 to 40 MPa. However, it is critical to understand this material's limits, such as its sensitivity to low temperatures, becoming fragile below −20°C, and susceptibility to expansion under UV light. PP also expands quickly when exposed to chlorinated solvents and aromatics (Shenoy and Patil 2010).

Despite these challenges, PP is widely used in the production of personalized 3D-printed prostheses for patients with bone fractures. This choice is primarily due to PP's remaining low weight and inherent rigidity qualities (Kim et al. 2022).

5.3.9 POLY-GLYCOLIC ACID

Poly-glycolic acid (PGA) emerges as a main synthetic polymer in the area of 3D scaffold creation due to its chemical versatility, simplicity to manufacture, and biocompatibility. The biodegradation of PGA produces glycolic acid monomer, an intermediate product that is quickly removed from the body via specific catabolic pathways, eventually resulting in carbon dioxide and water (Kim et al. 2022).

Furthermore, PGA's physical and mechanical qualities can be efficiently preserved using copolymers. This polymer is widely used in bone internal fixation devices and in the production of resorbable sutures. Notably, PGA's disintegrate products are non-toxic, making it suitable for a variety of biomedical applications (Ko et al. 2021).

5.3.10 POLYBUTYLENE TEREPHTHALATE

Polybutylene terephthalate (PBT) emerges as a biocompatible thermoplastic polyester that is widely employed in fused deposition modeling (FDM) printing methods. PBT is widely used in the biomedical field, both in vivo and in vitro, due to its good biocompatibility. It is known for its strong elasticity, ease of processing, and excellent strength and toughness (Chen et al. 2023).

PBT is important in tissue engineering because it enables the printing of bone scaffolds suited to canine trabecular bones and facilitates tissue regeneration. Furthermore, it is used as a filler in orthopedic procedures, demonstrating its versatility in biomedical applications (Chen et al. 2023).

However, it is critical to understand several limitations connected with PBT. Notably, PBTs degrade in aqueous conditions by hydrolysis or oxidation processes.

Furthermore, its high melting point of 225°C limits its use. Also, the nonbiodegradability of PBT causes the production of crystalline that remains in vivo, providing problems for its long-term use in biomedical applications (Chen et al. 2023).

5.3.11 POLYURETHANE

Polyurethane (PU) is a very promising flexible material known for its biodegradability, thermosetting properties, and great mechanical strength. PU stands out for its versatility, with variations available in both solvent-based and water-based forms (Chen et al. 2023).

Usually, solvent-based PU uses volatile organics as solvents, whereas water-based PU uses water as a solvent. This duality in solvent selection effects a variety of PU characteristics and applications. PU is extensively used in advanced printing processes such as stereolithography (SLA) and digital light processing (DLP), where its degradation profile is comparable to that of polylactic acid (PLA) (Chen et al. 2023).

PU has high printing resolution and great cytocompatibility, that make it ideal to develop complex structures with increased mechanical strength. PU is especially useful in cartilage tissue engineering, where it stimulates the production of chondrocytes, as well as bone construction and the development of scaffolds for muscle and nerve regeneration (Pugliese et al. 2021).

One of PU's most distinguishing characteristics is its excellent elastic properties, which allow it to resist repeated cycles of contraction and relaxation. This feature makes PU an excellent alternative for applications involving muscle tissue creation, where durability and robustness are critical (Pugliese et al. 2021).

5.3.12 POLYVINYL ALCOHOL

Polyvinyl alcohol (PVA) is a synthetic polymer made from vinyl alcohol and acetate monomers, which gives it a variety of useful properties. These monomers contribute to the biocompatibility, biodegradability, and semi-crystalline characteristics of PVA, making it an option for different biomedical applications (Pugliese et al. 2021).

Additionally, PVA is water soluble, distinguishing it from other polymer-based products. This property makes PVA appropriate for application in modern manufacturing procedures such as selective laser sintering (SLS), consequently improving its applicability in diverse biomedical applications (Pugliese et al. 2021).

PVA's tensile strength is comparable to that of human articular cartilage, indicating its potential for biomedical applications. Furthermore, PVA can form complex structures with excellent adhesion characteristics, making it an ideal matrix for stimulating bone cell ingrowth (Chen et al. 2023).

One of PVA's main advantages is its extraordinary hydrophilicity and chemical stability, which allow it to tolerate various pH and temperature conditions. Furthermore, its semi-crystalline form promotes the efficient flow of oxygen and nutrients to surrounding cells, creating an environment suitable to tissue regeneration (Camellia and Handoko 2022).

PVA's diverse characteristics make it useful for a variety of therapeutic treatments, including craniofacial defect correction and bone tissue engineering. However, it is important to highlight that PVA's water solubility might present difficulties in some applications, particularly where precise control over swelling behavior is required (Pugliese et al. 2021).

5.3.13 Polylactic-co-Glycolic Acid

Polylactic-co-glycolic acid (PLGA) is a polymer known for its consistent biodegradability and high cytocompatibility. These features make it an attractive candidate for a wide range of biomedical applications, including tissue engineering and regenerative medicine (Rocha et al. 2022; Elmowafy, Tiboni, and Soliman 2019).

One of the distinctive qualities of PLGA is its mechanical properties, which are like those of human calcium bone, making it osteoconductive. This property is crucial in supporting bone regeneration, as established in animal models and tissue-restoration systems (Rocha et al. 2022; Elmowafy, Tiboni, and Soliman 2019).

However, despite its promising properties, PLGA's hydrophobic characteristic limits its applicability. Furthermore, its linear structure contributes to low mechanical rigidity and a relatively fast disintegration rate, limiting its efficiency as a scaffold (Gentile et al. 2014; Elmowafy, Tiboni, and Soliman 2019).

When PLGA is inserted in vivo, its residues from decomposition have a high potential to cause inflammatory responses. The fragmentation of PLGA contaminants may increase this problem, possibly increasing the inflammatory response. Mixing PLGA with PCL is a promising method for reducing fracture and inflammatory reactions (Elmowafy, Tiboni, and Soliman 2019).

5.4   BIOINKS PROPERTIES FOR 3D PRINTING

Polymers have an important role in the development of biomaterials, providing a wide range of characteristics that have a significant impact on the properties of structures used in tissue engineering and regenerative medicine. These polymeric biomaterial properties include porosity, surface area, biocompatibility, biodegradability, and mechanical strength, all of which contribute uniquely to scaffold functionality and performance.

3D bioprinting is an innovative approach to generating complex tissues and organs with additive manufacturing techniques. Hydrogels are crucial to this process because they have porous architectures that can encapsulate and support a variety of cells and active chemicals. Whether using physical, chemical, or a mix of cross-linking processes, consistent printing properties such as density, viscosity, fluidity, and deformability are required for effective bioprinting. Furthermore, hydrogels must be biocompatible with organisms, meaning they are nontoxic, degradable, adhesive, and porous. As a result, a thorough understanding of the overall properties of 3D-printed hydrogels is necessary for evaluating their applicability for a variety of applications (Xie et al. 2023; Dell et al. 2022).

5.4.1 POROSITY

Porosity demonstrates a significant factor controlling many aspects of substructure behavior. Its importance extends to controlling cell proliferation, supporting the elimination of degraded compounds, and promoting vascularization in the scaffold structure. The material's porous structure helps to regulate nutrition flow and mechanical qualities, as well as the development and organization of the extracellular matrix. Optimal pore size ranges are required for certain tissue forms, with larger pore sizes promoting accelerated bone formation and vascularization processes and smaller pore sizes promoting neovascularization and fibroblast growth (Limon et al. 2023).

The observation of hydrogel structure, pore size, and porosity, using techniques such as scanning electron microscopy, provides information about printability and structural properties. Hydrogels with high porosity are necessary for oxygen and nutrient delivery, cell motility, and angiogenesis. Imaging techniques such as microcomputed tomography and X-ray propagation-based imaging allow for the reconstruction of 3D structures and investigation of porosity, which improves our understanding of hydrogel printability (Rodríguez-Rego et al. 2022).

5.4.2 SURFACE AREA

Surface area is another crucial aspect influencing scaffold function. A bigger and more accessible surface area promotes cell anchoring and proliferation, both of which are critical for restoring or maintaining tissue or organ functions. Biocompatibility, which is closely related to surface area, refers to a material's capacity to sustain biological activity while avoiding undesirable reactions. It is determined by a complex interaction of elements such as polymer chemistry, morphology, and structure, with some polymers, such as PLA, PLGA, and PGA, having particularly good biocompatibility characteristics (Tejada Jacob et al. 2022).

Printing accuracy, or the degree of fidelity to a CAD plan, is an important characteristic in bioprinting. This accuracy consists of the characteristics of the printed samples, such as diameter, uniformity, angle, and printed area. Maintaining appropriate structural and shape accuracy in 3D bioprinting of hydrogels is difficult due to the materials' intrinsic flow behavior and weak mechanical qualities, especially when generating large clinical-scale tissue constructions. It is an important indicator of the bioprinting capabilities of bioinks, with strategies such as adding cationic modified silica nanoparticles into anionic polymer mixes proving helpful in improving printing fidelity (Rodríguez-Rego et al. 2022; He et al. 2016).

5.4.3 BIODEGRADABILITY AND BIOCOMPATIBILITY

Biodegradability is a crucial factor in scaffold design, since it allows for regulated disintegration over time to generate space for developed tissues. This property improves both drug delivery and tissue engineering systems, enabling scaffold dissolution and tissue regeneration. Polymer biodegradation occurs by the breaking of susceptible hydrolytic or enzymatic bonds and is regulated by a number of parameters, including chemical structure, molecular weight, and hydrophilicity/hydrophobicity. Nonbiodegradable polymers, on the other hand, provide long-term support and durability, making them viable alternatives for applications that require scaffold stability over time (Echeverria Molina, Malollari, and Komvopoulos 2021).

In practical applications, 3D-bioprinted hydrogels are biocompatible, biodegradable, and cost-effective. These hydrogels are frequently coupled with cells, growth hormones, and other compounds to form appropriate microenvironments for a variety of biological purposes. The improved cell survival, proliferation, and differentiation inside hydrogel matrices highlight their promise for dynamic and individualized biological structures, paving the door for advances in tissue engineering and regenerative medicine (Temirel, Hawxhurst, and Tasoglu 2021).

5.4.4 MECHANICAL AND RHEOLOGICAL PROPERTIES

Mechanical qualities are also important in scaffold performance because they determine how well the scaffold can tolerate stresses and strains during tissue growth and regeneration. These mechanical properties together determine the scaffold's mechanical integrity and robustness, which are critical for tissue regeneration processes and drug delivery. Rheological and mechanical characteristics such as maximum strain, elastic modulus, and tensile strength are important parameters determined by pore access, size, form, and volume (Barrulas and Corvo 2023).

The rheological properties of 3D bioprinting hydrogels, such as viscosity, shear thinning, and thixotropic behavior, are critical for print quality, processing, and cell viability. Flow rheometry is a measurement technique that provides insights into the viscosity of bioinks at different shear rates. The impact of electric charge on biological printing is visible in its effects on bioink viscosity and shear rate. Hydrogel precursors frequently display non-Newtonian behavior, which results in nonlinear shear stress - shear rate curves with low viscosity. While high viscosity at moderate shear rates allows bioinks to maintain stable structures after printing, excessive viscosity could affect cell survival and function, necessitating an accurate equilibrium between printing accuracy and cellular compatibility (Wang et al. 2021; Bercea 2023).

The hydrogel 3D printing process is usually separated into three stages: the structural change of the bioink from a liquid to a gel state during extrusion, the formation of printing layers and layer adhesion on the substrate to print multilayer structures, and the self-supporting stage of structural recovery. Rheological research helps to evaluate printing behavior over a variety of process parameters, allowing hydrogels to be identified in different states. Furthermore, the elastic modulus, which affects the deformation of 3D structures under strain, influences printing ability, with hydrogels with adaptable mechanical characteristics being particularly useful in obtaining shape fidelity (Herrada-Manchón, Fernández, and Aguilar 2023; Wang et al. 2021; He et al. 2016).

Research to improve the stability and mechanical integrity of 3D bioprinted hydrogels show promise for applications such as cartilage regeneration. Strategies incorporating the modulation of fibrinogen material, modification, and cross-linking procedures have been effective in improving cytocompatibility and allowing cell embedding for tissue development. Furthermore, hydrogels protect cells from shear stress–induced damage during printing, creating an optimal environment for cell adhesion, proliferation, and migration. As researchers continue to improve the properties of printable, high-fidelity, and biocompatible 3D printing scaffolds, the sector is getting closer to satisfying the broad clinical needs of tissue regeneration and beyond (Agarwal et al. 2023; Gao, Kim, and Gao 2021).

5.5   3D BIOPRINTING TECHNOLOGIES

There are many methods for manufacturing hydrogels using bioprinting technology, each with its own set of benefits and applications. There are several 3D bioprinting methods, significant approaches include inkjet bioprinting, extrusion bioprinting, laser-assisted bioprinting, stereolithography bioprinting, suspension bioprinting, and digital 3D bioprinting (Xie et al. 2023; Lima et al. 2022; Ramiah et al. 2020).

As bioprinting technology advances, the overriding goal remains consistent: to assure cell viability, printing fidelity, and scaffold lifetime in order to meet clinical demands for tissue and organ engineering. The potential of 3D biological printing is expanding with continual innovation and study, opening up previously unexplored possibilities in regenerative medicine and tissue engineering (Ramadan and Zourob 2020; Kantaros 2022; Jiang, Mei, and Zhao 2021).

5.5.1   INKJET-BASED BIOPRINTING

Inkjet technology is a great discovery in the field of printing, characterized by its precision in producing droplets by volume range and its ability to jet thousands of these droplets each second. While inkjet technology initially became popular in traditional printing applications such as graphics and document reproduction, it has quickly expanded, finding significant utility in the pharmaceutical industry (Uddin, Hassan, and Douroumis 2022).

One of the most interesting aspects of inkjet technology is its non-contact printing process, which has resulted in considerable advances in bioprinting. Despite previous printing methods involving direct contact with the substrate, inkjet-based printing allows for the deposition of ingredients without contact with the substrate, providing a precise and efficient method of protecting sensitive biological components (Rider et al. 2018).

In the context of bioprinting, inkjet technology provides remarkable versatility, notably in manipulating cell densities within printed structures. Inkjet printers can create gradients of cell populations inside a single structure by accurately altering factors such as droplet density or size, allowing for the development of complex tissue models with diverse cellular compositions (Mani et al. 2022; Rider et al. 2018; Gillispie et al. 2020).

In essence, inkjet-based bioprinting is a revolutionary method to tissue engineering, providing unparalleled control and precision in the creation of functioning tissue structures. As research in this field progresses, inkjet technology is expected to play an increasingly important role in the development of advanced biomedical solutions, propelling innovation and advancement in regenerative medicine and customized healthcare (Mani et al. 2022).

5.5.2 EXTRUSION BIOPRINTING

Extrusion bioprinting has become a highly effective and widely recognized 3D printing process in the fields of tissue engineering and biological manufacturing. The operating premise is to load bioink into a syringe barrel and then extrude it through a micronozzle needle. This simple and efficient approach has various benefits, including affordability, cost-effectiveness, and adaptability, making it a great choice for tissue engineering and biological manufacturing (Liu et al. 2022; Kačarević et al. 2018).

One of extrusion bioprinting's elementary advantages is its capacity to provide for the continuous deposition of various bioinks in a controlled method. Extrusion bioprinting, which quickly alternates between multiple bioink reservoirs, enables the fabrication of heterogeneous tissue structures with diverse cellular compositions and configurations (Davoodi et al. 2020).

Extrusion bioprinting has several advantages, but it also has some limitations. One of the most significant challenges is bioink viscosity. The viscosity of the bioink can have a considerable impact on its extrudability and printability, necessitating the optimization of formulation parameters for appropriate printing results. Furthermore, the intrinsic limitations of extrusion-based printing processes, such as low resolution and limited droplet size control, make it difficult to develop high-fidelity structures with complex characteristics (Chen et al. 2023; Derakhshanfar et al. 2018).

Moreover, while extrusion bioprinting offers a viable means of fabricating tissue-like structures, concerns regarding cell viability and functionality persist. The mechanical forces exerted during the extrusion process can subject cells to shear stress and other forms of mechanical damage, potentially compromising their viability and biological activity. As such, strategies to enhance cell survival and maintain functionality within the printed constructs are critical areas of focus for ongoing research and development efforts in extrusion bioprinting (Malekpour and Chen 2022).

Considering these obstacles, extrusion bioprinting techniques require innovation and improvement. Advances in bioink formulation, the nozzle design, and printing settings can resolve current challenges.

5.5.3 LASER-ASSISTED BIOPRINTING

Laser-induced forward transfer bioprinting, an innovative method that eliminates the need for nozzles, provides great precision, automation, and cell survival rates. This method uses laser technology to enable in-situ printing of bioink, promoting tissue regeneration and the development of precisely complex tissue models. The inherent benefits of laser-based bioprinting include the capacity to produce high-resolution printing, precise control over droplet deposition, and minimal mechanical stress on the printed cells, resulting in enhanced cell survivability and performance (Chang and Sun 2023).

In addition, laser bioprinting technology has enormous potential for expanding the applications of regenerative medicine and tissue engineering by allowing for the development of complex tissue architectures with precision and accuracy. Researchers and clinicians can create customized tissue constructs specific to individual patients' unique anatomical and physiological characteristics, for personalized regenerative therapies and organ replacement alternatives (Jiang, Mei, and Zhao 2021).

However, despite its potential, laser-induced forward transfer bioprinting has some obstacles. The intrinsic complexity of the laser source is one of the most critical challenges in terms of system design, operation, and maintenance. The intricate structure of laser-based bioprinting systems necessitates precise instrumentation, careful calibration, and meticulous control over numerous variables to ensure optimal performance and reproducibility (Chang and Sun 2023; Shakil Arman et al. 2023).

Furthermore, using laser technology in bioprinting systems adds challenges related to safety, regulatory compliance, and cost-effectiveness. The procurement and maintenance of high-powered laser systems require significant financial and technical resources, limiting access to this advanced technology for many researchers and organizations (Chang and Sun 2023).

However, these difficulties can be resolved and the potential of laser-induced forward transfer bioprinting can be explored with the contribution of regular improvements in laser technology and inventive bioprinting techniques. Researchers can use laser-based bioprinting to improve tissue engineering and regenerative medicine by resolving technological limitations, improving printing parameters, and improving system accessibility.

5.5.4 Stereolithography Bioprinting

Stereolithography is an advanced additive manufacturing technique that uses rapid prototyping technology to create complex objects with precision, dimensional accuracy, and quality. With the use of photopolymerization techniques, stereolithography makes it possible to precisely cure liquid resin materials, which are exposed to ultraviolet (UV) light, so that 3D objects can be constructed layer by layer (Kushwaha et al. 2022).

Recent advances in 3D bioprinting have made it possible to print solid hydrogel models quickly and effectively with little cell damage or distortion due to exact control over photopolymerization conditions. Despite conventional techniques, which frequently need extended exposure to environmental stresses and severe curing conditions, hydrogel stereolithography allows hydrogel-based constructions to be quickly created while maintaining the viability and functionality of encapsulated cells (Grigoryan et al. 2021).

Fast hydrogel stereolithography's success is mainly due to its capacity to precisely control the photopolymerization process, optimizing variables such as light intensity, exposure duration, and resin composition to provide the required printing results. Through the adjustment of these parameters, researchers can modify the process of printing according to the particular requirements of different hydrogel compositions, providing the cell survival, structural stability, and mechanical characteristics in the printed structures (Anandakrishnan et al. 2021).

Furthermore, stereolithography's fast prototyping capabilities make it possible to create complex geometries with speed and accuracy. This capability offers new opportunities for the design and manufacturing of personalized organ models, tissue scaffolds, and biomedical devices that are appropriate to each patient's particular demands. Fast hydrogel stereolithography, whether used in drug delivery systems, regenerative medicine applications, or in vitro tissue modeling, has great potential to advance biomedical research and clinical practice (Anandakrishnan et al. 2021).

5.6   APPLICATION OF 3D BIOPRINTING

3D bioprinting has emerged as a very promising technology that efficiently integrates cells with specialized hydrogel inks to create complex tissue-like structures using precise layer-by-layer manufacturing techniques. This technique accurately simulates the environment of tissues and cells, suggesting great potential for tissue engineering applications in repair and reconstruction. Within the biomedical field, the discussion is mostly focused on the many different uses of bone, skin, and cardiovascular tissue engineering, demonstrating the diversity and range of impact offered by this innovative technology.

5.6.1   BONE TISSUE

Bone is a complex structure made up of hierarchical tissue structures interconnected with mineralized collagen fibers, a vascular network, and other components. While bones have extraordinary regenerating powers and can repair tiny cracks and fractures on themselves, bigger fractures in bones of more than 2 mm provide major challenges because self-repair mechanisms become insufficient. Large imperfections demand bone regeneration with personalized implants to restore both form and function. However, typical hydrogels have difficulties with accurately adjusting the interior of bone structure and the distribution of growth factors, resulting in the development of new methodologies such as 3D bioprinting (Alves et al. 2023; Yazdanpanah et al. 2022).

The use of 3D bioprinting techniques to process biomaterials, including cells, has enormous potential to improve bone tissue engineering through facilitating the construction of complex functional 3D structures. Additionally, cross-linked hydrogel inks that contain calcium ions, such as sodium alginate and GelMA, are increasingly of interest (Tolmacheva, Bhattacharyya, and Noh 2024; Patrocinio et al. 2023; Maresca et al. 2023).

In addition, the interaction between biological components, specifically collagen and supportive hydrogels have been used to increase hardness. For example, bone marrow mesenchymal stem cells demonstrate osteogenic development within agarose collagen hydrogels, which have low hardness and promote cell expansion and branching (Tolmacheva, Bhattacharyya, and Noh 2024; Patrocinio et al. 2023; Maresca et al. 2023).

Despite these advances, significant problems persist, particularly in mimicking the mechanical characteristics of real bone and obtaining high mineralization and varied cell proliferation. While hydrogel-loaded stem cells show promise for encouraging bone regeneration using 3D bioprinting, more studies are needed to create novel materials and procedures that can satisfy these specifications (Tolmacheva, Bhattacharyya, and Noh 2024; Patrocinio et al. 2023; Maresca et al. 2023).

5.6.2 Skin Tissue

The skin is the body's main barrier against external factors such as bacteria, parasites, temperatures, ultraviolet (UV) radiation, and transpiration of water. Despite its protective function, skin disorders are the fourth most common nonfatal disease worldwide, affecting around one-third of the global population. The natural process of wound healing consists of several complex actions, including hemostasis, inflammation, proliferation, and extracellular matrix remodeling. While typical wound treatments give protection against contamination, they require periodic replacements and often restrict mobility in joints, providing significant challenges for patients (Gushiken et al. 2021).

Hydrogels have emerged as the preferred bioinks for 3D bioprinting due to their biocompatibility and degradability. There has been substantial study on the use of 3D-printed hydrogels as biological scaffolding for treating skin injuries (Maresca et al. 2023).

In addition, researchers have derived endothelial cells from induced pluripotent stem cells, fibroblasts, pericytes, and human keratinocytes to produce skin-equivalent tissues with varying physiological complexities, including human epidermis and full-thickness skin equivalents for drug screening. These skin models have layered structural characteristics in the dermis and epidermis and mimic the physiological function of the skin barrier, providing useful insights into disease causes as well as pharmacological efficacy and toxicity testing (Gushiken et al. 2021).

To summarize, 3D-printed hydrogels, whether used as drug delivery or cell transporters, have enormous potential in the treatment of skin injuries. While hyaluronic acid and sodium alginate are commonly used as hydrogel inks in skin tissue engineering, developing a skin bioprint remains difficult due to its complex structure and extensions. As a result, there is an important requirement to investigate novel biological hydrogel inks and printing technologies.

5.6.3 CARDIOVASCULAR TISSUE

The cardiovascular system, which includes the heart, blood arteries, and lymphatic systems, is critical for life support. Unfortunately, cardiovascular disorders continue in the most prevalent diseases around the world.

While vascular transplants are currently used to treat serious cardiovascular problems, autografts are frequently inefficient and offer a risk of secondary consequences for patients. As a result, several technologies have developed to replicate the complex vascular systems, with 3D bioprinting emerging as an important instrument to develop vascular biomimetic structures. Its benefits include precise control over vascular development, scalability in manufacturing, and reproducibility (Kang et al. 2023).

In addition, 3D-printed hydrogels have demonstrated potential as cardiac patches for the treatment of cardiovascular disorders. Researchers used novel techniques including aerosol jet printing to manufacture 2D titanium carbide MXene–hydrogel composites for human cardiac patches. Methacrylate gelatin/polyethylene glycol diacrylate/alginate, cross-linked by light exposure, offer a promising additional treatment for heart valve dysfunction. Furthermore, a 3D-bioprinted hydrogel scaffold prepared using a two-step cross-linking method that combines physical cross-linking of alginate with chemical crosslinking of GelMA exhibits precise control over microfiber anisotropic structure and promotes the formation of endothelialized human myocardial models (Kang et al. 2023).

Despite these advances, the application of 3D-bioprinted patient-specific cardiac patches for heart failure treatment is still at the experimental stage. Developing heart-specific bioinks that meet cardiac tissue's distinct cell heterogeneity and functional requirements remains a challenge. The careful balance between fidelity and printability is critical, as hydrogel instability may affect printing precision. Solving these obstacles and utilizing modern 3D bioprinting technology will advance the use of bioprinting in cardiovascular treatment.

REFERENCES

Agarwal, Kirti, Varadharajan Srinivasan, Viney Lather, Deepti Pandita, and Kirthanashri S. Vasanthan. 2023. "Insights of 3D Bioprinting and Focusing the Paradigm Shift towards 4D Printing for Biomedical Applications." *Journal of Materials Research* 38 (1): 112–41. https://doi.org/10.1557/s43578-022-00524-2.

Ahmadi Soufivand, Anahita, Jessica Faber, Jan Hinrichsen, and Silvia Budday. 2023. "Multilayer 3D Bioprinting and Complex Mechanical Properties of Alginate-Gelatin Mesostructures." *Scientific Reports* 13 (1): 1–14. https://doi.org/10.1038/s41598-023-38323-2.

Alves, Bruno C., Renato S. de Miranda, Barbara M. Frigieri, Debora A. P. C. Zuccari, Marcia R. de Moura, Fauze A. Aouada, and Ruís C. Tokimatsu. 2023. "A 3D Printing Scaffold Using Alginate/Hydroxyapatite for Application in Bone Regeneration." *Materials Research* 26: 1–7. https://doi.org/10.1590/1980-5373-MR-2023-0051.

Amni, C. Marwan, S. Aprilia, and E. Indarti. 2021. "Current Research in Development of Polycaprolactone Filament for 3D Bioprinting: A Review." *IOP Conference Series: Earth and Environmental Science* 926 (1). https://doi.org/10.1088/1755-1315/926/1/012080.

Anandakrishnan, N., Z. Guo, H. Ye, Z. Chen, K. I. Mentkowski, J. K. Lang, N. Rajabian, S. T. Andreadis, et al. 2021. "Fast Stereolithography Printing of Large-Scale Biocompatible Hydrogel Models." *Advanced Healthcare Materials* 10: 2002103.

Nagaraj, Anushree, Alaitz Etxabide Etxeberria, Rafea Naffa, Ghada Zidan, and Ali Seyfoddin. 2022. "3D-Printed Hybrid Collagen/GelMA Hydrogels for Tissue Engineering Applications." *Biology* 11 (11): 1561.

Askari, Mohsen, Moqaddaseh Afzali Naniz, Monireh Kouhi, Azadeh Saberi, Ali Zolfagharian, and Mahdi Bodaghi. 2021. "Recent Progress in Extrusion 3D Bioprinting of Hydrogel Biomaterials for Tissue Regeneration: A Comprehensive Review with Focus on Advanced Fabrication Techniques." *Biomaterials Science* 9 (3): 535–73. https://doi.org/10.1039/d0bm00973c.

Axpe, Eneko, and Michelle L. Oyen. 2016. "Applications of Alginate-Based Bioinks in 3D Bioprinting." *International Journal of Molecular Sciences* 17 (12). https://doi.org/10.3390/ijms17121976.

Barrulas, Raquel V., and Marta C. Corvo. 2023. "Rheology in Product Development: An Insight into 3D Printing of Hydrogels and Aerogels †." *Gels* 9 (12). https://doi.org/10.3390/gels9120986.

Bercea, Maria. 2023. "Rheology as a Tool for Fine-Tuning the Properties of Printable Bioinspired Gels." *Molecules* 28 (6). https://doi.org/10.3390/molecules28062766.

Bupphathong, Sasinan, Carlos Quiroz, Wei Huang, Pei Feng Chung, Hsuan Ya Tao, and Chih Hsin Lin. 2022. "Gelatin Methacrylate Hydrogel for Tissue Engineering Applications—A Review on Material Modifications." *Pharmaceuticals* 15 (2). https://doi.org/10.3390/ph15020171.

Caliari, Steven R., and Jason A. Burdick. 2016. "A Practical Guide to Hydrogels for Cell Culture." *Nature Methods* 13 (5): 405–14. https://doi.org/10.1038/nmeth.3839.

Camellia, Tea, and Fauzi Handoko. 2022. "Synthesis and Physicochemical Properties of Poly (Vinyl) Alcohol Nanocomposites Reinforced with Nanocrystalline." https://www.inbar.int/resources/inbar_publications/trade-overview-2020-bamboo-and-rattan-commodities-in-the-international-market/.

Castañeda-Rodríguez, Samanta, Maykel González-Torres, Rosa María Ribas-Aparicio, María Luisa Del Prado-Audelo, Gerardo Leyva-Gómez, Eda Sönmez Gürer, and Javad Sharifi-Rad. 2023. "Recent Advances in Modified Poly (Lactic Acid) as Tissue Engineering Materials." *Journal of Biological Engineering* 17 (1): 1–20. https://doi.org/10.1186/s13036-023-00338-8.

Cavallo, Aida, Tamer Al Kayal, Angelica Mero, Andrea Mezzetta, Lorenzo Guazzelli, Giorgio Soldani, and Paola Losi. 2023. "Fibrinogen-Based Bioink for Application in Skin Equivalent 3D Bioprinting." *Journal of Functional Biomaterials* 14 (9). https://doi.org/10.3390/jfb14090459.

Chang, Jinlong, and Xuming Sun. 2023. "Laser-Induced Forward Transfer Based Laser Bioprinting in Biomedical Applications." *Frontiers in Bioengineering and Biotechnology* 11 (August): 1–11. https://doi.org/10.3389/fbioe.2023.1255782.

Chen, Heming, Quan Shi, Hengtao Shui, Peng Wang, Qiang Chen, and Zhiyong Li. 2021. "Degradation of 3D-Printed Porous Polylactic Acid Scaffolds Under Mechanical Stimulus." *Frontiers in Bioengineering and Biotechnology* 9 (October): 1–9. https://doi.org/10.3389/fbioe.2021.691834.

Chen, Qizhou, Yi Qi, Yuwei Jiang, Weiyan Quan, Hui Luo, Kefeng Wu, Sidong Li, and Qianqian Ouyang. 2022. "Progress in Research of Chitosan Chemical Modification Technologies and Their Applications." *Marine Drugs* 20 (8). https://doi.org/10.3390/md20080536.

Chen, X. B., A. Fazel Anvari-Yazdi, X. Duan, A. Zimmerling, R. Gharraei, N. K. Sharma, S. Sweilem, and L. Ning. 2023. "Biomaterials / Bioinks and Extrusion Bioprinting." *Bioactive Materials* 28 (May): 511–36. https://doi.org/10.1016/j.bioactmat.2023.06.006.

Davoodi, Elham, Einollah Sarikhani, Hossein Montazerian, Samad Ahadian, Marco Costantini, Wojciech Swieszkowski, Stephanie Michelle Willerth, et al. 2020. "Extrusion and Microfluidic-Based Bioprinting to Fabricate Biomimetic Tissues and Organs." *Advanced Materials Technologies* 5 (8). https://doi.org/10.1002/admt.201901044.

Dell, Annika C., Grayson Wagner, Jason Own, and John P. Geibel. 2022. "3D Bioprinting Using Hydrogels: Cell Inks and Tissue Engineering Applications." *Pharmaceutics* 14 (12). https://doi.org/10.3390/pharmaceutics14122596.

Derakhshanfar, Soroosh, Rene Mbeleck, Kaige Xu, Xingying Zhang, Wen Zhong, and Malcolm Xing. 2018. "3D Bioprinting for Biomedical Devices and Tissue Engineering: A Review of Recent Trends and Advances." *Bioactive Materials* 3 (2): 144–56. https://doi.org/10.1016/j.bioactmat.2017.11.008.

Dong, Chanjuan, and Yonggang Lv. 2016. "Application of Collagen Scaffold in Tissue Engineering: Recent Advances and New Perspectives." *Polymers* 8 (2): 1–20. https://doi.org/10.3390/polym8020042.

Echeverria Molina, Maria I., Katerina G. Malollari, and Kyriakos Komvopoulos. 2021. "Design Challenges in Polymeric Scaffolds for Tissue Engineering." *Frontiers in Bioengineering and Biotechnology* 9 (June): 1–29. https://doi.org/10.3389/fbioe.2021.617141.

Elmowafy, Enas M., Mattia Tiboni, and Mahmoud E. Soliman. 2019. Biocompatibility, Biodegradation and Biomedical Applications of Poly(Lactic Acid)/Poly(Lactic-Co-Glycolic Acid) Micro and Nanoparticles. *Journal of Pharmaceutical Investigation* 49. https://doi.org/10.1007/s40005-019-00439-x.

Fang, Wenzhuo, Ming Yang, Meng Liu, Yangwang Jin, Yuhui Wang, Ranxing Yang, Ying Wang, Kaile Zhang, and Qiang Fu. 2023. "Review on Additives in Hydrogels for 3D Bioprinting of Regenerative Medicine: From Mechanism to Methodology." *Pharmaceutics* 15 (6). https://doi.org/10.3390/pharmaceutics15061700.

Farshidfar, Nima, Siavash Iravani, and Rajender S. Varma. 2023. "Alginate-Based Biomaterials in Tissue Engineering and Regenerative Medicine." *Marine Drugs* 21 (3). https://doi.org/10.3390/md21030189.

Freeman, Sebastian, Stefano Calabro, Roma Williams, Sha Jin, and Kaiming Ye. 2022. "Bioink Formulation and Machine Learning-Empowered Bioprinting Optimization." *Frontiers in Bioengineering and Biotechnology* 10 (June): 1–16. https://doi.org/10.3389/fbioe.2022.913579.

Gao, Qiqi, Byoung Soo Kim, and Ge Gao. 2021. "Advanced Strategies for 3D Bioprinting of Tissue and Organs Analogs Using Alginate Hydrogel Bioinks." *Marine Drugs* 19 (12). https://doi.org/10.3390/md19120708.

Gentile, Piergiorgio, Valeria Chiono, Irene Carmagnola, and Paul V. Hatton. 2014. "An Overview of Poly(Lactic-Co-Glycolic) Acid (PLGA)-Based Biomaterials for Bone Tissue Engineering." *International Journal of Molecular Sciences* 15 (3): 3640–59. https://doi.org/10.3390/ijms15033640.

Ghosh, Rudra Nath, Joseph Thomas, B. R. Vaidehi, N. G. Devi, Akshitha Janardanan, Pramod
    K. Namboothiri, and Mathew Peter. 2023. "An Insight into Synthesis, Properties
    and Applications of Gelatin Methacryloyl Hydrogel for 3D Bioprinting." *Materials
    Advances* 4 (22): 5496–529. https://doi.org/10.1039/d3ma00715d.
Gibney, Rory, Jennifer Patterson, and Eleonora Ferraris. 2021. "High-Resolution Bioprinting
    of Recombinant Human Collagen Type Iii." *Polymers* 13 (17). https://doi.org/10.3390/
    polym13172973.
Gillispie, Gregory J., Albert Han, Meryem Uzun-Per, John Fisher, Antonios G. Mikos,
    Muhammad Khalid Khan Niazi, James J. Yoo, Sang Jin Lee, and Anthony Atala. 2020.
    "The Influence of Printing Parameters and Cell Density on Bioink Printing Outcomes."
    Tissue Engineering - Part A 26 (23–24): 1349–58. https://doi.org/10.1089/ten.tea.2020
    .0210.
Gonzalez-Fernandez, Tomas, Alejandro J. Tenorio, Kevin T. Campbell, Eduardo A. Silva,
    and J. Kent Leach. 2021. "Alginate-Based Bioinks for 3D Bioprinting and Fabrication
    of Anatomically Accurate Bone Grafts." *Tissue Engineering - Part A* 27 (17–18): 1168–
    81. https://doi.org/10.1089/ten.tea.2020.0305.
Gopinathan, Janarthanan, and Insup Noh. 2018. "Recent Trends in Bioinks for 3D Printing."
    Biomaterials Research 22 (1): 1–15. https://doi.org/10.1186/s40824-018-0122-1.
Grigoryan, Bagrat, Daniel W. Sazer, Amanda Avila, Jacob L. Albritton, Aparna Padhye,
    Anderson H. Ta, Paul T. Greenfield, Don L. Gibbons, and Jordan S. Miller. 2021.
    "Development, Characterization, and Applications of Multi-Material Stereolithography
    Bioprinting." *Scientific Reports* 11 (1): 1–13. https://doi.org/10.1038/s41598-021-82102
    -w.
Guo, Chuang, Jiacheng Wu, Yiming Zeng, and Hong Li. 2023. "Construction of 3D
    Bioprinting of HAP/Collagen Scaffold in Gelation Bath for Bone Tissue Engineering."
    Regenerative Biomaterials 10 (August). https://doi.org/10.1093/rb/rbad067.
Gushiken, Lucas Fernando Sérgio, Fernando Pereira Beserra, Jairo Kenupp Bastos,
    Christopher John Jackson, and Cláudia Helena Pellizzon. 2021. "Cutaneous Wound
    Healing: An Update from Physiopathology to Current Therapies." *Life* 11 (7): 1–15.
    https://doi.org/10.3390/life11070665.
Hauptstein, Julia, Thomas Böck, Michael Bartolf-Kopp, Leonard Forster, Philipp
    Stahlhut, Ali Nadernezhad, Gina Blahetek, et al. 2020. "Hyaluronic Acid-Based
    Bioink Composition Enabling 3D Bioprinting and Improving Quality of Deposited
    Cartilaginous Extracellular Matrix." *Advanced Healthcare Materials* 9 (15): 1–15.
    https://doi.org/10.1002/adhm.202000737.
Hauser, Peter Viktor, Hsiao Min Chang, Masaki Nishikawa, Hiroshi Kimura, Norimoto
    Yanagawa, and Morgan Hamon. 2021. "Bioprinting Scaffolds for Vascular Tissues and
    Tissue Vascularization." *Bioengineering* 8 (11). https://doi.org/10.3390/bioengineer
    ing8110178.
He, Yong, Feifei Yang, Haiming Zhao, Qing Gao, Bing Xia, and Jianzhong Fu. 2016.
    "Research on the Printability of Hydrogels in 3D Bioprinting." *Scientific Reports* 6:
    1–13. https://doi.org/10.1038/srep29977.
Herrada-Manchón, Helena, Manuel Alejandro Fernández, and Enrique Aguilar. 2023.
    "Essential Guide to Hydrogel Rheology in Extrusion 3D Printing: How to Measure It
    and Why It Matters?" *Gels* 9 (7). https://doi.org/10.3390/gels9070517.
Ji, Shen, and Murat Guvendiren. 2017. "Recent Advances in Bioink Design for 3D Bioprinting
    of Tissues and Organs." *Frontiers in Bioengineering and Biotechnology* 5 (APR): 1–8.
    https://doi.org/10.3389/fbioe.2017.00023.
Jiang, Wei, Haiying Mei, and Shuyan Zhao. 2021. "Applications of 3D Bio-Printing in Tissue
    Engineering and Biomedicine." *Journal of Biomedical Nanotechnology* 17 (6): 989–
    1006. https://doi.org/10.1166/jbn.2021.3078.

Kačarević, Željka P., Patrick M. Rider, Said Alkildani, Sujith Retnasingh, Ralf Smeets, Ole Jung, Zrinka Ivanišević, and Mike Barbeck. 2018. "An Introduction to 3D Bioprinting: Possibilities, Challenges and Future Aspects." *Materials* 11 (11). https://doi.org/10.3390/ma11112199.

Kang, Moon Sung, Jinju Jang, Hyo Jung Jo, Won Hyeon Kim, Bongju Kim, Heoung Jae Chun, Dohyung Lim, and Dong Wook Han. 2023. "Advances and Innovations of 3D Bioprinting Skin." *Biomolecules* 13 (1). https://doi.org/10.3390/biom13010055.

Kantaros, Antreas. 2022. "3D Printing in Regenerative Medicine: Technologies and Resources Utilized." *International Journal of Molecular Sciences* 23 (23). https://doi.org/10.3390/ijms232314621.

Kapusetti, Govinda, Namdev More, and Mounika Choppadandi. 2019. "Introduction to Ideal Characteristics and Advanced Biomedical Applications of Biomaterials." In *Biomedical Engineering and Its Applications in Healthcare*, 171–204. Springer.

Kim, Sunjung, Sai Yalla, Sagar Shetty, and Noah J. Rosenblatt. 2022. "3D Printed Transtibial Prosthetic Sockets: A Systematic Review." *PLoS ONE* 17 (10 October): 1–19. https://doi.org/10.1371/journal.pone.0275161.

Kniebs, Caroline, Franziska Kreimendahl, Marius Köpf, Horst Fischer, Stefan Jockenhoevel, and Anja Lena Thiebes. 2020. "Influence of Different Cell Types and Sources on Pre-Vascularisation in Fibrin and Agarose–Collagen Gels." *Organogenesis* 16 (1): 14–26. https://doi.org/10.1080/15476278.2019.1697597.

Ko, Han Seung, Sangwoon Lee, Doyoung Lee, and Jae Young Jho. 2021. "Mechanical Properties and Bioactivity of Poly(Lactic Acid) Composites Containing Poly(Glycolic Acid) Fiber and Hydroxyapatite Particles." *Nanomaterials* 11 (1): 1–13. https://doi.org/10.3390/nano11010249.

Kohane, Daniel S., and Robert Langer. 2008. "Polymeric Biomaterials in Tissue Engineering." *Pediatric Research* 63 (5): 487–91. https://doi.org/10.1203/01.pdr.0000305937.26105.e7.

Kress, Sebastian, Johannes Baur, Christoph Otto, Natalie Burkard, Joris Braspenning, Heike Walles, Joachim Nickel, and Marco Metzger. 2018. "Evaluation of a Miniaturized Biologically Vascularized Scaffold in Vitro and in Vivo." *Scientific Reports* 8 (1): 1–13. https://doi.org/10.1038/s41598-018-22688-w.

Kushwaha, Amanendra K., Md Hafizur Rahman, David Hart, Branden Hughes, Diego Armando Saldana, Carson Zollars, Dipen Kumar Rajak, and Pradeep L. Menezes. 2022. "Fundamentals of Stereolithography: Techniques, Properties, and Applications." In *Tribology of Additively Manufactured Materials*. Elsevier.

Lazaridou, Maria, Dimitrios N. Bikiaris, and Dimitrios A. Lamprou. 2022. "3D Bioprinted Chitosan-Based Hydrogel Scaffolds in Tissue Engineering and Localised Drug Delivery." *Pharmaceutics* 14 (9). https://doi.org/10.3390/pharmaceutics14091978.

Lee Kuen Yong, and David J. Mooney. 2012. "Alginate: Properties and Biomedical Applications." *Progress in Polymer Science (Oxford)* 37 (1): 106–26. https://doi.org/10.1016/j.progpolymsci.2011.06.003.

Li, Na, Rui Guo, and Zhenyu Jason Zhang. 2021. "Bioink Formulations for Bone Tissue Regeneration." *Frontiers in Bioengineering and Biotechnology* 9 (February): 1–17. https://doi.org/10.3389/fbioe.2021.630488.

Li, Xiaorui, Fuyin Zheng, Xudong Wang, Xuezheng Geng, Shudong Zhao, Hui Liu, Dandan Dou, Yubing Leng, Lizhen Wang, and Yubo Fan. 2022. "Biomaterial Inks for Extrusion-Based 3D Bioprinting: Property, Classification, Modification, and Selection." *International Journal of Bioprinting* 9 (2). https://doi.org/10.18063/IJB.V9I2.649.

Li Xinda, Boxun Liu, Ben Pei, Jianwei Chen, Dezhi Zhou, Jiayi Peng, Xinzhi Zhang, Wang Jia, and Tao Xu. 2020. "Inkjet Bioprinting of Biomaterials." *Chemical Reviews* 120 (19): 10793–833. https://doi.org/10.1021/acs.chemrev.0c00008.

Li Ying, Xueqin Zhang, Xin Zhang, Yuxuan Zhang, and Dan Hou. 2023. "Recent Progress of the Vat Photopolymerization Technique in Tissue Engineering: A Brief Review of Mechanisms, Methods, Materials, and Applications." *Polymers* 15 (19). https://doi.org /10.3390/polym15193940.

Lima, Tainara de P. L., Caio Augusto d. A. Canelas, Viktor O. C. Concha, Fernando A. M. da Costa, and Marcele F. Passos. 2022. "3D Bioprinting Technology and Hydrogels Used in the Process." *Journal of Functional Biomaterials* 13 (4): 1–18. https://doi.org /10.3390/jfb13040214.

Limon, Shah M., Connor Quigley, Rokeya Sarah, and Ahasan Habib. 2023. "Advancing Scaffold Porosity through a Machine Learning Framework in Extrusion Based 3D Bioprinting." *Frontiers in Materials* 10 (February): 1–13. https://doi.org/10.3389/fmats .2023.1337485.

Liu, Na, Xiaopei Zhang, Qingxia Guo, Tong Wu, and Yuanfei Wang. 2022. "3D Bioprinted Scaffolds for Tissue Repair and Regeneration." *Frontiers in Materials* 9 (July): 1–17. https://doi.org/10.3389/fmats.2022.925321.

López-Marcial, Gabriel R., Anne Y. Zeng, Carlos Osuna, Joseph Dennis, Jeannette M. García, and Grace D. O'Connell. 2018. "Agarose-Based Hydrogels as Suitable Bioprinting Materials for Tissue Engineering." *ACS Biomaterials, Science e Enginnering.*

Lukin, Izeia, Itsasne Erezuma, Lidia Maeso, Jon Zarate, Martin Federico Desimone, Taleb H. Al-Tel, Alireza Dolatshahi-Pirouz, and Gorka Orive. 2022. "Progress in Gelatin as Biomaterial for Tissue Engineering." *Pharmaceutics* 14 (6): 1–19. https://doi.org/10 .3390/pharmaceutics14061177.

Lyu, Su Ping, and Darrel Untereker. 2009. "Degradability of Polymers for Implantable Biomedical Devices." *International Journal of Molecular Sciences* 10 (9): 4033–65. https://doi.org/10.3390/ijms10094033.

Ma, Xuanyi, Justin Liu, Wei Zhu, Min Tang, Natalie Lawrence, Claire Yu, Maling Gou, and Shaochen Chen. 2018. "3D Bioprinting of Functional Tissue Models for Personalized Drug Screening and in Vitro Disease Modeling." *Advanced Drug Delivery Reviews* 132: 235–51. https://doi.org/10.1016/j.addr.2018.06.011.

Maiz-Fernández, Sheila, Leyre Pérez-álvarez, Unai Silván, José Luis Vilas-Vilela, and Senentxu Lanceros-Méndez. 2022. "PH-Induced 3D Printable Chitosan Hydrogels for Soft Actuation." *Polymers* 14 (3). https://doi.org/10.3390/polym14030650.

Malekpour, Ali, and Xiongbiao Chen. 2022. "Printability and Cell Viability in Extrusion-Based Bioprinting from Experimental, Computational, and Machine Learning Views." *Journal of Functional Biomaterials* 13 (2). https://doi.org/10.3390/jfb13020040.

Mallakpour, Shadpour, Fariba Sirous, and Chaudhery Mustansar Hussain. 2021. "Current Achievements in 3D Bioprinting Technology of Chitosan and Its Hybrids." *New Journal of Chemistry* 45 (24).

Mani, Mohan Prasath, Madeeha Sadia, Saravana Kumar Jaganathan, Ahmad Zahran Khudzari, Eko Supriyanto, Syafiqah Saidin, Seeram Ramakrishna, Ahmad Fauzi Ismail, and Ahmad Athif Mohd Faudzi. 2022. "A Review on 3D Printing in Tissue Engineering Applications." *Journal of Polymer Engineering* 42 (3): 243–65. https://doi .org/10.1515/polyeng-2021-0059.

Maresca, Jamie A., Derek C. DeMel, Grayson A. Wagner, Colin Haase, and John P. Geibel. 2023. "Three-Dimensional Bioprinting Applications for Bone Tissue Engineering." *Cells* 12 (9). https://doi.org/10.3390/cells12091230.

Mattos, Bruno D., André L. Misso, Pedro H. G. De Cademartori, Edson A. De Lima, Washington L. E. Magalhães, and Darci A. Gatto. 2014. "Properties of Polypropylene Composites Filled with a Mixture of Household Waste of Mate-Tea and Wood Particles." *Construction and Building Materials* 61: 60–68. https://doi.org/10.1016/j .conbuildmat.2014.02.022.

Melo, Bruna A. G. de, Yasamin A. Jodat, Elisa M. Cruz, Julia C. Benincasa, Su Ryon Shin, and Marimelia A. Porcionatto. 2020. "Strategies to Use Fibrinogen as Bioink for 3D Bioprinting Fibrin-Based Soft and Hard Tissues." *Acta Biomaterialia* 117: 60–76. https://doi.org/10.1016/j.actbio.2020.09.024.

Mendoza-Cerezo, Laura, Jesús M. Rodríguez-Rego, Antonio Macías-García, Alfonso C. Marcos-Romero, and Antonio Díaz-Parralejo. 2023. "Evolution of Bioprinting and Current Applications." *International Journal of Bioprinting* 9 (4). https://doi.org/10.18063/ijb.742.

Merazzo, Karla J., Ander García Díez, Carmen R. Tubio, Juan Carlos Manchado, Ramón Malet, Marc Pérez, Pedro Costa, and Senentxu Lanceros-Mendez. 2023. "Acrylonitrile Butadiene Styrene-Based Composites with Permalloy with Tailored Magnetic Response." *Polymers* 15 (3): 1–19. https://doi.org/10.3390/polym15030626.

Miller, Jordan S., Colette J. Shen, Wesley R. Legant, Jan D. Baranski, Brandon L. Blakely, and Christopher S. Chen. 2010. "Bioactive Hydrogels Made from Step-Growth Derived PEG-Peptide Macromers." *Biomaterials* 31 (13): 3736–43. https://doi.org/10.1016/j.biomaterials.2010.01.058.

Mirdamadi, Eman, Narine Muselimyan, Priyanka Koti, Huda Asfour, and Narine Sarvazyan. 2019. "Agarose Slurry as a Support Medium for Bioprinting and Culturing Freestanding Cell-Laden Hydrogel Constructs." *3D Printing and Additive Manufacturing* 6 (3): 158–64. https://doi.org/10.1089/3dp.2018.0175.

Mora Boza, Ana, Malgorzata K. Wlodarczyk-Biegun, Aránzazu Del Campo, Blanca Vázquez-Lasal, and Julio San Román. 2019. "Chitosan-Based Inks: 3D Printing and Bioprinting Strategies to Improve Shape Fidelity, Mechanical Properties, and Biocompatibility of 3D Scaffolds." *Biomecánica* 27: 7–16. https://doi.org/10.5821/sibb.27.1.9199.

Naghieh, Saman, Mohammad Reza Karamooz-Ravari, M. D. Sarker, Eva Karki, and Xiongbiao Chen. 2018. "Influence of Crosslinking on the Mechanical Behavior of 3D Printed Alginate Scaffolds: Experimental and Numerical Approaches." *Journal of the Mechanical Behavior of Biomedical Materials* 80: 111–18.

Nayak, Vasudev Vivekanand, Nick Tovar, Doha Khan, Angel Cabrera Pereira, Dindo Q. Mijares, Marcus Weck, Alejandro Durand, et al. 2023. "3D Printing Type 1 Bovine Collagen Scaffolds for Tissue Engineering Applications—Physicochemical Characterization and In Vitro Evaluation." *Gels* 9 (8). https://doi.org/10.3390/gels9080637.

Neves, Mariana Isabel, Lorenzo Moroni, and Cristina Carvalho Barrias. 2020. "Modulating Alginate Hydrogels for Improved Biological Performance as Cellular 3D Microenvironments." *Frontiers in Bioengineering and Biotechnology* 8 (June). https://doi.org/10.3389/fbioe.2020.00665.

Nishimura, Shinichiro, Osamu Kohgo, Keisuke Kurita, and Hiroyoshi Kuzuhara. 1991. "Chemospecific Manipulations of a Rigid Polysaccharide: Syntheses of Novel Chitosan Derivatives with Excellent Solubility in Common Organic Solvents by Regioselective Chemical Modifications." *Macromolecules* 24: 4745–48.

Noh, Insup, Nahye Kim, Hao Nguyen Tran, Jaehoo Lee, and Chibum Lee. 2019. "3D Printable Hyaluronic Acid-Based Hydrogel for Its Potential Application as a Bioink in Tissue Engineering." *Biomaterials Research* 23 (1): 1–9. https://doi.org/10.1186/s40824-018-0152-8.

Osidak, Egor Olegovich, Vadim Igorevich Kozhukhov, Mariya Sergeevna Osidak, and Sergey Petrovich Domogatsky. 2020. "Collagen as Bioink for Bioprinting: A Comprehensive Review." *International Journal of Bioprinting* 6 (3): 1–10. https://doi.org/10.18063/IJB.V6I3.270.

Patrocinio, David, Victor Galván-Chacón, J. Carlos Gómez-Blanco, Sonia P. Miguel, Jorge Loureiro, Maximiano P. Ribeiro, Paula Coutinho, J. Blas Pagador, and Francisco M. Sanchez-Margallo. 2023. "Biopolymers for Tissue Engineering: Crosslinking, Printing Techniques, and Applications." *Gels.* https://search.proquest.com/docview/63288937 ?accountid=13042%250Ahttp://oxfordsfx.hosted.exlibrisgroup.com/oxford?url_ver =Z39.88-2004&rft_val_fmt=info:ofi/fmt:kev:mtx:journal&genre=article&sid=ProQ: ProQ%253Aeric&atitle=Techniques+and+Applications&title=Ba.

Pereira, Inês, Maria J. Lopez-Martinez, Aranzazu Villasante, Clelia Introna, Daniel Tornero, Josep M. Canals, and Josep Samitier. 2023. "Hyaluronic Acid-Based Bioink Improves the Differentiation and Network Formation of Neural Progenitor Cells." *Frontiers in Bioengineering and Biotechnology* 11 (March): 1–15. https://doi.org/10.3389/fbioe .2023.1110547.

Perez-Puyana, Victor, Mercedes Jiménez-Rosado, Alberto Romero, and Antonio Guerrero. 2020. "Polymer-Based Scaffolds for Soft-Tissue Engineering." *Polymers* 12: 1566.

Pitto-Barry, Anaïs, and Nicolas P. E. Barry. 2014. "Pluronic® Block-Copolymers in Medicine: From Chemical and Biological Versatility to Rationalisation and Clinical Advances." *Polymer Chemistry* 5 (10): 3291–97. https://doi.org/10.1039/c4py00039k.

Pugliese, Raffaele, Benedetta Beltrami, Stefano Regondi, and Christian Lunetta. 2021. "Polymeric Biomaterials for 3D Printing in Medicine: An Overview." *Annals of 3D Printed Medicine* 2. https://doi.org/10.1016/j.stlm.2021.100011.

Ramadan, Qasem, and Mohammed Zourob. 2020. "3D Bioprinting at the Frontier of Regenerative Medicine, Pharmaceutical, and Food Industries." *Frontiers in Medical Technology* 2 (January): 1–19. https://doi.org/10.3389/fmedt.2020.607648.

Ramiah, Previn, Lisa C. du Toit, Yahya E. Choonara, Pierre P. D. Kondiah, and Viness Pillay. 2020. "Hydrogel-Based Bioinks for 3D Bioprinting in Tissue Regeneration." *Frontiers in Materials* 7 (April): 1–13. https://doi.org/10.3389/fmats.2020.00076.

Rider, Patrick, Željka Perić Kačarević, Said Alkildani, Sujith Retnasingh, and Mike Barbeck. 2018. "Bioprinting of Tissue Engineering Scaffolds." *Journal of Tissue Engineering* 9. https://doi.org/10.1177/2041731418802090.

Rocha, Cátia Vieira, Victor Gonçalves, Milene Costa da Silva, Manuel Bañobre-López, and Juan Gallo. 2022. "PLGA-Based Composites for Various Biomedical Applications." *International Journal of Molecular Sciences* 23 (4). https://doi.org/10.3390/ ijms23042034.

Rodríguez-Rego, Jesús M., Laura Mendoza-Cerezo, Antonio Macías-García, Juan P. Carrasco-Amador, and Alfonso C. Marcos-Romero. 2022. "Methodology for Characterizing the Printability of Hydrogels." *International Journal of Bioprinting* 9 (2): 280–91. https:// doi.org/10.18063/IJB.V9I2.667.

Rojas-Murillo, Juan Antonio, Mario A. Simental-Mendía, Nidia K. Moncada-Saucedo, Paulina Delgado-Gonzalez, José Francisco Islas, Jorge A. Roacho-Pérez, and Elsa N. Garza-Treviño. 2022. "Physical, Mechanical, and Biological Properties of Fibrin Scaffolds for Cartilage Repair." *International Journal of Molecular Sciences* 23 (17). https://doi.org/10.3390/ijms23179879.

Roy, Jagadish C., Fabien Salaun, Stéphane Giraund, and Ada Ferri. 2017. "Solubility of Chitin: Solvents, Solution Behaviors and Their Related Mechanisms." In *Solubility of Polysaccharides*. InTech.

Sahoo, Deepti Rekha, and Trinath Biswal. 2021. "Alginate and Its Application to Tissue Engineering." *SN Applied Sciences* 3 (1). https://doi.org/10.1007/s42452-020-04096-w.

Salati, Mohammad Amin, Javad Khazai, Amir Mohammad Tahmuri, Ali Samadi, Ali Taghizadeh, Mohsen Taghizadeh, Payam Zarrintaj, et al. 2020. "Agarose-Based Biomaterials: Opportunities and Challenges in Cartilage Tissue Engineering." *Polymers* 12 (5): 1–15. https://doi.org/10.3390/POLYM12051150.

Sanz-Horta, Raúl, Ana Matesanz, Alberto Gallardo, Helmut Reinecke, José Luis Jorcano, Pablo Acedo, Diego Velasco, and Carlos Elvira. 2023. "Technological Advances in Fibrin for Tissue Engineering." *Journal of Tissue Engineering* 14. https://doi.org/10.1177/20417314231190288.

Sekar, Muthu Parkkavi, Shruthy Suresh, Allen Zennifer, Swaminathan Sethuraman, and Dhakshinamoorthy Sundaramurti. 2023. "Hyaluronic Acid as Bioink and Hydrogel Scaffolds for Tissue Engineering Applications." *ACS Biomaterials Science and Engineering* 9 (6): 3134–59.

Shakil Arman, Md, Ben Xu, Andrew Tsin, and Jianzhi Li. 2023. "Laser-Induced Forward Transfer (LIFT) Based Bioprinting of the Collagen I with Retina Photoreceptor Cells." *Manufacturing Letters* 35: 477–84. https://doi.org/10.1016/j.mfglet.2023.07.005.

Shenoy, M. A., and Mrinalini Patil. 2010. "Studies in Reduction of Molecular Weight of Polypropylene." *Polymer Science – Series B* 52 (3–4): 174–83. https://doi.org/10.1134/S1560090410030073.

Sikorski, Dominik, Karolina Gzyra-Jagieła, and Zbigniew Draczyński. 2021. "The Kinetics of Chitosan Degradation in Organic Acid Solutions." *Marine Drugs* 19 (5): 1–16. https://doi.org/10.3390/md19050236.

Stafin, Krzysztof, Paweł Śliwa, and Marek Piątkowski. 2023. "Towards Polycaprolactone-Based Scaffolds for Alveolar Bone Tissue Engineering: A Biomimetic Approach in a 3D Printing Technique." *International Journal of Molecular Sciences* 24 (22). https://doi.org/10.3390/ijms242216180.

Stepanovska, Jana, Monika Supova, Karel Hanzalek, Antonin Broz, and Roman Matejka. 2021. "Collagen Bioinks for Bioprinting: A Systematic Review of Hydrogel Properties, Bioprinting Parameters, Protocols, and Bioprinted Structure Characteristics." *Biomedicines* 9 (9). https://doi.org/10.3390/biomedicines9091137.

Tejada Jacob, Guillermo, Verónica E. Passamai, Sergio Katz, Guillermo R. Castro, and Vera Alvarez. 2022. "Hydrogels for Extrusion-Based Bioprinting: General Considerations." *Bioprinting* 27 (May). https://doi.org/10.1016/j.bprint.2022.e00212.

Temirel, Mikail, Christopher Hawxhurst, and Savas Tasoglu. 2021. "Shape Fidelity of 3D-Bioprinted Biodegradable Patches." *Micromachines* 12 (2). https://doi.org/10.3390/mi12020195.

Tolmacheva, Nelli, Amitava Bhattacharyya, and Insup Noh. 2024. "Calcium Phosphate Biomaterials for 3D Bioprinting in Bone Tissue Engineering." *Biomimetics* 9 (2): 1–24. https://doi.org/10.3390/biomimetics9020095.

Uddin, Md Jasim, Jasmin Hassan, and Dennis Douroumis. 2022. "Thermal Inkjet Printing: Prospects and Applications in the Development of Medicine." *Technologies* 10 (5): 10–14. https://doi.org/10.3390/technologies10050108.

Wang, Qingbo, Oskar Backman, Markus Nuopponen, Chunlin Xu, and Xiaoju Wang. 2021. "Rheological and Printability Assessments on Biomaterial Inks of Nanocellulose/Photo-Crosslinkable Biopolymer in Light-Aided 3D Printing." *Frontiers in Chemical Engineering* 3 (September): 1–13. https://doi.org/10.3389/fceng.2021.723429.

Wang, Xiaohong. 2019. "Advanced Polymers for Three-Dimensional (3D) Organ Bioprinting." *Micromachines* 10 (12): 1–25. https://doi.org/10.3390/mi10120814.

Wang, Xiaohong, Qiang Ao, Xiaohong Tian, Jun Fan, Hao Tong, Weijian Hou, and Shuling Bai. 2017. "Gelatin-Based Hydrogels for Organ 3D Bioprinting." *Polymers* 9 (9). https://doi.org/10.3390/polym9090401.

Wenger, Lukas, Carsten P. Radtke, Eva Gerisch, Max Kollmann, Christof M. Niemeyer, Kersten S. Rabe, and Jürgen Hubbuch. 2022. "Systematic Evaluation of Agarose- and Agar-Based Bioinks for Extrusion-Based Bioprinting of Enzymatically Active Hydrogels." *Frontiers in Bioengineering and Biotechnology* 10 (November): 1–17. https://doi.org/10.3389/fbioe.2022.928878.

Xie, Mengbo, Jingjing Su, Shengxi Zhou, Jingan Li, and Kun Zhang. 2023. "Application of Hydrogels as Three-Dimensional Bioprinting Ink for Tissue Engineering." *Gels* 9 (2). https://doi.org/10.3390/gels9020088.

Yasin, Aqeela, Ying Ren, Jingan Li, Yulong Sheng, Chang Cao, and Kun Zhang. 2022. "Advances in Hyaluronic Acid for Biomedical Applications." *Frontiers in Bioengineering and Biotechnology* 10 (July): 1–12. https://doi.org/10.3389/fbioe.2022 .910290.

Yazdanpanah, Zahra, James D. Johnston, David M. L. Cooper, and Xiongbiao Chen. 2022. "3D Bioprinted Scaffolds for Bone Tissue Engineering: State-Of-The-Art and Emerging Technologies." *Frontiers in Bioengineering and Biotechnology* 10 (April). https://doi.org/10.3389/fbioe.2022.824156.

Yusof, Wan Roslina Wan, Nur Yusra Farzana Awang, Muhammad Affuwan Azhar Laile, Juzaili Azizi, Awang Ahmad Sallehin Awang Husaini, Azman Seeni, Lee D. Wilson, and Sumiyyah Sabar. 2023. "Chemically Modified Water-Soluble Chitosan Derivatives: Modification Strategies, Biological Activities, and Applications." *Polymer-Plastics Technology and Materials* 62 (16): 2182–220.

6 4D Printing

6.1 SMART MATERIAL PRINTING

Four-dimensional (4D) printing emerged as an innovative technology during the additive manufacturing revolution, transcending the horizons previously outlined by conventional 3D printing. While 3D printing brought about a transformation in how we conceive and produce objects, 4D printing incorporates a temporal dimension, starting an era where printed constructs are no longer static but dynamic and capable of adapting in response to external stimuli.

4D printing is nothing more than an extension of 3D printing technology, adding the dimension of time to the equation. While 3D printing creates 3Dw objects layer-by-layer, 4D printing introduces the capability for these objects to change their shape, properties, or function over time in response to external stimuli such as heat, humidity, or other environmental factors.

The process often involves the use of smart materials or programmable materials that can respond to specific stimuli. These materials may be designed to expand, contract, or undergo other changes in shape or function based on external stimuli (Figure 6.1).

The unique aspect of 4D printing unfolds after the completion of the physical printing. The subsequent steps involve the activation of smart materials, triggering dynamic transformations in the printed object over time. These transformations can range from structural changes to alterations in fundamental physical properties, such as shape, rigidity, or even the color of the object.

As previously mentioned, the 4D printing process typically involves the use of smart or programmable materials. These materials can be polymers or composites with the ability to respond to specific stimuli such as heat, light, humidity, or other environmental conditions. The materials' response may include changes in shape, rigidity, color, or other physical properties (Borse and Shende 2023).

At the heart of this innovation lies the careful selection of smart, programmable, and stimuli-sensitive materials. The 4D printing process begins with the 3D design of the desired object, before proceeding to careful material selection, and culminates in the printing of 3D layers, similar to the 3D printing process.

6.1.1 TYPES OF STIMULI IN 4D PRINTING

In 4D printing, various types of stimuli can be employed to induce changes in printed structures over time. Stimulus play a fundamental role in 4D printing as they are responsible for inducing the desired changes in the printed structures over time. The

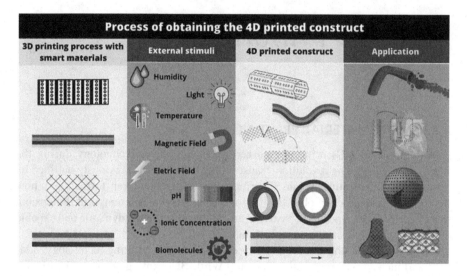

FIGURE 6.1 Types of external stimuli to obtain the 4D printed construct for biomedical and pharmaceutical applications.

ability to control and program these changes enables the creation of dynamic and adaptive materials and devices with a wide range of applications.

6.1.1.1 Physical Signal

6.1.1.1.1 Humidity

Some polymers are responsive to changes in humidity, leading to swelling or contraction. Water and humidity were the first external stimuli employed in 4D printing. Materials sensitive to water or humidity are of significant interest due to their ubiquitous presence and extensive applications. By utilizing water as an external stimulus, the structure can be deformed underwater and restored to its original shape after drying. However, it is crucial to precisely control the degree of expansion/contraction of the moisture-sensitive material during the transition to preserve the integrity of the printed structure.

For this type of stimulus, it is necessary to use hygroscopic polymers, which absorb water and, thus, undergo changes in their shape, volume, or other physical properties. When exposed to water or moisture, these materials can expand, contract, or undergo some other form of controlled transformation.

6.1.1.1.2 Temperature

Changes in temperature can trigger responses in thermosensitive polymers. When temperature serves as the external stimulus, the shape-changing mechanism is referred to as unrestricted thermomechanism. This method requires two temperature levels: T_h (above the glass transition temperature (T_g) of the smart material) and T_L (below T_g). The desired shape is achieved when the printed structure is cooled to T_L. Subsequently, the structure is heated to T_H to restore its original shape (Megdich,

Habibi, and Laperrière 2023). The primary categories of temperature-responsive polymers frequently employed in 4D printing applications include: (i) shape memory polymers and (ii) responsive polymer solutions (Hoogenboom 2014).

6.1.1.1.3   Light

The use of light as a stimulus for response in 4D printing offers various advantages and innovative possibilities. This approach, often referred to as photopolymerization, involves the use of light-sensitive materials that can change shape or properties in response to exposure to light of certain characteristics, such as intensity, wavelength, or lighting pattern. As a result of light exposure, the polymer responds by altering its structure, returning to its pre-programmed original shape or assuming a new form.

Some advantages of using light as a stimulus include precision, speed, remote control, and versatility. Light can be precisely controlled to create complex exposure patterns, enabling the production of intricate and detailed structures. In addition, photopolymerization can occur rapidly, allowing for shorter production times compared to other 4D printing methods.

6.1.1.1.4   Pressure

Mechanical pressure or stress can induce responses in piezoelectric or rheological polymers. Pressure stimulation in 4D printing involves the utilization of materials or structures that respond to changes in pressure to achieve dynamic transformations over time. By incorporating pressure-sensitive materials or mechanisms into the printing process, such as pneumatic actuators or smart materials, it becomes possible to create objects that can deform, change shape, or exhibit other desired behaviors in response to varying levels of pressure. This capability opens up opportunities for applications in fields such as soft robotics, adaptive structures, and biomedical devices, where pressure-responsive behavior is advantageous for functionality and performance.

6.1.1.1.5   Magnetic

Magnetic fields can influence polymers containing magnetic particles. The action of the magnetic field is achieved by introducing magnetic particles into the polymeric system. Under the influence of the magnetic field, the magnetic particles convert the energy from the external magnetic field into thermal energy through the mechanism of loss. Among magnetic particles, Fe_3O_4 nanoparticles are easy to synthesize on a large scale, as they are low cost and have good biocompatibility.

6.1.1.1.6   Electric Fields

Application of an electric current can influence conductive polymers. Some materials are sensitive to electric fields, altering their properties in response to the presence of an electric charge. These materials are known as electroresponsive or electroactive. Similar to light, the electric field can also be used as a stimulus in remote control. When used as a stimulus, the electric field generates a resistive impulse to fill a shape-memory polymer with conductive filler. The use of electric fields in 4D printing can have various applications, ranging from the creation of biomimetic devices that move in response to electric stimuli to adaptable electronic components that change their properties in specific environments.

Typically, these devices have been limited to single trigger responses, whereas in the natural environment, devices are exposed to multiple stimuli simultaneously. Responsiveness to multiple stimuli in printed objects has been gaining attention, and understanding how the material behaves under different stimuli is crucial (Cremonini et al. 2023). This ability to respond to multiple external stimuli offers remarkable versatility in the creation of 4D objects, enabling an even broader range of adaptive applications and functionalities. However, the complexity of designing and controlling these materials increases when multiple stimuli are incorporated, requiring special care to ensure the integrity and desired functionality of the construct.

6.1.1.2   Chemical Signal

6.1.1.2.1   pH

Exposure to specific chemicals or pH changes can trigger responses in chemoresponsive polymers. Polymers sensitive to pH variations can undergo structural or property changes in response to alterations in the surrounding pH environment (Tran et al. 2022; Mukhopadhyay et al. 2014). These pH-responsive polymers contain functional groups that ionize or de-ionize depending on the pH level of the solution they are exposed to. This ionization process can lead to changes in the polymer's swelling behavior, solubility, or mechanical properties (Tran et al. 2022; Dai, Ravi, and Tam 2008; Muzaffar et al. 2020). In 4D printing, pH-responsive polymers can be incorporated into printing materials or used as support structures. By controlling the pH of the printing environment, it's possible to trigger shape changes or other dynamic responses in the printed objects. This pH-responsive behavior opens up possibilities for creating smart structures that can adapt to different pH conditions, making them potentially useful in applications such as drug delivery systems, sensing devices, or environmental sensors.

6.1.1.2.2   Ionic

Ionic stimulation in 4D printing involves the use of materials that respond to changes in the ionic concentration of the surrounding environment. These materials, known as ionic hydrogels, can undergo alterations in their properties, such as volume, stiffness, or water retention capacity, in response to variations in ion concentration in the solution. Hydrogels containing ionic groups can interact with ions in the solution, causing changes in electrostatic repulsion between the polymeric chains and, consequently, in the gel's properties (Kang et al. 2007; Huang et al. 2017). This can lead to reversible changes in the hydrogel structure, such as expansion or contraction as a response to changes in ion concentration. Ionic stimulation offers an intriguing approach to 4D printing as it allows for the control of the properties of printed structures by manipulating the ionic composition of the surrounding environment.

6.1.1.3   Biological Signal

Biological stimulation in 4D printing involves the use of materials or techniques that respond to biological cues or stimuli to achieve dynamic transformations over time.

These biological cues can include factors such as biological small molecules or bio-macromolecules such as glucose, enzymes, nucleic acids, polypeptides, and proteins present in the surrounding environment (Hu, Katti, and Gu 2014; E. Song, da Costa, and Choi 2017; Adams, Malkoc, and La Belle 2018).

6.2 SMART POLYMERS

Polymers with shape memory are smart materials that play a key role in 4D printing, with the ability to recover their permanent shapes from one or sometimes multiple programmed temporary shapes when an appropriate stimulus is applied (Table 6.1). These transformative properties of smart materials generate 4D-printed structures with responsiveness, self-detection, self-repair, shape memory, multifunctionality, and self-adaptability (Mao et al. 2015; W. Zhao et al. 2023).

Due to the capability of these smart materials to detect environmental changes and react according to a predefined sequence, they emerge as promising candidates for applications where spontaneous conformational change is required. Additionally, they can be chemically tuned to achieve biocompatibility and biodegradability and, therefore, have been extensively studied for biomedical and pharmaceutical applications. The 4D printed structure can be obtained by using a memory polymer or a mixture of them. The choice of polymers will depend on the functionality and application of the structure obtained.

6.2.1 Types of Structures

The material structures are divided into monomaterial and multimaterial structures. The choice between monomaterial and multimaterial structures will depend on the specific needs of the application, the desired complexity, and good levels of control during the manufacturing process.

Monomaterials: Provide good levels of control and are simple to manufacture, making them easier to implement. However, they may have limitations in terms of the diversity of dynamic responses.

Multimaterials: Allow for a greater diversity of responses and functionalities but involve additional challenges in printing and controlling interactions between different materials.

6.2.1.1 Single-Material Structures

Monomaterials refer to structures printed using a single type of material (Alshebly et al. 2022; Megdich, Habibi, and Laperrière 2023). 4D printing with monomaterials typically involves a single polymer or material that exhibits specific properties in response to external stimuli such as water, temperature, light, etc. (Liu et al. 2021; Alshebly et al. 2022). The single-material structure utilizes a single smart material with a gradient distribution. This anisotropy can produce shape-changing behaviors such as bending and twisting and are simpler to control and print as they involve only one type of material.

TABLE 6.1

Type of Stimulus, Printer, and Application in Obtaining Constructs from 4D Printing

Signal	Stimulus Type	Polymer	Printer	Application	Reference(s)
Physical	Electric Field	PANI	Direct ink writing	Energy and electric devices at micro-nano scale	(Wang et al. 2018)
		Combine plain PLA with conductive PLA	FDM	Electric device	(Mitkus, Cerbe, and Sinapius 2022)
	Humidity	GelMA	Extrusion	Tissue engineering	(Zhao, Lai, and Wang 2021)
		PHG	Stereolithography	Regenerative medicine	(Jamal et al. 2013)
		PVA	FDM	Gastric retention	(Melocchi et al. 2019)
	Light	pNIPAM and PEG	Extrusion	Controlled drug release	(Zu et al. 2022)
		CA-PLA-PEG	FDM	Tissue repair	(Luo et al. 2023)
		PEG-norbornene	Extrusion	Scaffolds and tissue culture	(Miksch et al. 2022)
	Magnetic Field	Iron oxide particles were incorporated to the crosslinked PVA	Extrusion	-	(Chuayprakong, Wanamonkol, and Khayandee 2020)
		pNIPAM, PEG and iron oxide nanoparticles	Extrusion	Delivery approach	(Choi et al. 2023)
		ALG, methylcellulose and iron oxide	Extrusion	Soft robots in medicine and biomedical engineering	(Siminska-Tanny et al. 2022)
	Pressure	PLA	FDM	Stress-absorbers	(Barletta, Gisario, and Mehrpouya 2021)
	Temperature	LCE	Ink writing	Tissue engineering	(Qiu et al. 2023)
		PEGDA	DLP	Microneedle	(Han et al. 2020)
		PLA	FDM	Smart textiles	(Leist et al. 2017)
		PLA	FDM	Vascular stents	(Wu et al. 2018)
		PLA and PCL	Ink writing	Tracheal scaffolds	(Pandey, Mohol, and Kandi 2022)
		PLA and PEA for shape-memory with added barium titanate	Deposition via electric poling-assisted	Biomedical implants	(Bodkhe and Ermanni 2020)
		PLA and PU	FDM printer equipped with two nozzles	-	(Rahmatabadi et al. 2023)
		PLA/PCL-based CBPU	FDM	Bio-tissue engineering, soft robotics, and intlligent sensors	(Song et al. 2022)
		pNIPAM	Silicon templates produced by Photolithography	Tissue engineering scaffold	(Ozturk et al. 2009)
		PVA/(PVA-MA)$_2$-g-PNIPAM	DLP	Soft actuators and robots	(Hua et al. 2021)
		VeroWhite and Tangoblack	Jet spraying before UV curing	Biomedical	(Mao et al. 2015)

(Continued)

TABLE 6.1 (CONTINUED)

Type of Stimulus, Printer, and Application in Obtaining Constructs from 4D Printing

Signal	Stimulus Type	Polymer	Printer	Application	Reference(s)
Chemical	Ionic	ALG and and methacrylated type I collagen	Extrusion	Artificial corneal structures	(Isaacson, Swioklo, and Connon 2018)
		ALG and methylcellulose	Extrusion	tissue engineering, biomedical device and soft robotics fields	(Lai et al. 2021)
		ALG, methylcellulose, and iron oxide	Extrusion	Soft robots in medicine and biomedical engineering	(Siminska - Stanny et al. 2022)
	pH	Carbon nanotube-based and polyaniline nanowire-based ink: 1) glucose is catalyzed and 2) platinum nanoparticles catalyze hydrogen peroxide	Inkjet	Kit for glucose measurement	(Song, Da Costa, and Choi 2017)
		Cross-linking PHEAA-co-PMVK with a bifunctional hydroxylamine	FDM	Biomedical application	(Nadgorny et al. 2018)
		Collagen	Drop-on-demand inkjet	Skin engineering	(Lee et al. 2014)
		PMAA	Soft-lithography	Oral delivery	(He, Guan, and Lee 2006)
Biological	Glucose	Graphene polylactic acid filament	FDM	Sensitive glucose detection	(Adams, Malkoc, and La Belle 2018)
		Carbon nanotube-based and polyaniline nanowire-based ink: 1) glucose is catalyzed and 2) platinum nanoparticles catalyze hydrogen peroxide	Inkjet	Kit for glucose measurement	(Song, Da Costa, and Choi 2017)
	Enzymes	GelMA microswimmers	Stereolithography	Microrobots medicine	(Wang et al. 2018)

Note: Alginate (Alg); Bio-polyurethane material (CBPU); Digital light processing (DLP); Fused deposition modeling (FDM); Gelatin methacryloyl (GelMA); Liquid crystal elastomers (LCE); Polyaniline (PANI); Polycaprolactone (PCL); Polyesteramide (PEA); poly (ethylene glycol) (PEG); Poly(ethyleneglycol) diacrylate (PEGDA); Polylactic acid (PLA); Poly(l-lactic acid) (PLLA); Poly(N-isopropylacrylamide) (pNIPAM); poly(methyacrylic acid) (PMAA); poly(n-hydroxy-ethyl acrylamide-co-methyl vinyl ketone) (PHEAA-co-PMVK); Polystyrene-b-poly(2-vinyl pyridine) (PS-b-P2VP), Polyurethane (PU) and Poly(vinyl alcohol) (PVA).

6.2.1.2 Multi-Material Structures

Multimaterials refer to printed structures using two or more types of polymers (Tibbits 2014). The multimaterial structure can be made from different smart materials or a combination of smart and conventional materials with distinct properties. Each material can respond to specific stimuli, providing a broader range of responses and functionalities. They are more complex due to the need to control multiple materials and their interactions.

Three types of multimaterial structures are mentioned in the 4D printing literature: uniform distribution, gradient distribution, and special patterns. Composite structure is an important type of special pattern (Megdich, Habibi, and Laperrière 2023). This technique is used to enhance the shape recoverability and mechanical properties of the material.

6.2.2 TYPES OF POLYMERS

In 4D printing, a variety of polymers can be used depending on the specific properties desired for the final object and responsiveness to external stimuli.

6.2.2.1 Polylactic Acid (PLA)

PLA is an optically active substance. Additionally, it presents important characteristics for obtaining a 4D structure in the biomedical field, as it has good biodegradability. In vivo, PLA can be hydrolyzed by hydrolase to convert the polymer into a monomer and metabolized into water and carbon dioxide. PLA is known for its biocompatibility and is derived from renewable sources such as corn starch or sugarcane. This makes it an attractive choice for medical and environmentally conscious applications in 4D printing (Wang and Li 2020; Mehrpouya et al. 2021).

Although PLA itself is not a polymer sensitive to external stimuli, it can be combined with active materials that respond to stimuli such as light, temperature, or water. In some 4D printing applications, PLA can be used as support or inert structure for active components. For example, in a composite structure, PLA can provide the support structure while active materials, such as light-sensitive polymers, are printed on it. Due to being a stiffer polymer, it has a lower tendency to deform over some other materials used in 4D printing. This can be advantageous for maintaining the shape and dimensional stability of structures during the printing process and over time. Given its biocompatibility and biodegradability, an attractive application of 4D printing with PLA is in the medical field, especially in surgical settings (Leist et al. 2017; Wu et al. 2018).

The use of PLA in obtaining 4D-printed constructs sparks interest in various fields, particularly in biomedical engineering. Due to its excellent shape memory properties, biocompatibility, low cost, and easy processing PLA emerges as an attractive material. However, this material can be enhanced by introducing materials and approaches such as composites that combine PLA with nanomaterials to achieve innovative designs and create objects that change shape in response to different external stimuli.

6.2.2.2   Polycaprolactone (PCL)

Like PLA, PCL is a shape memory polymer and can be combined with active materials that respond to external stimuli such as light, temperature, or water. This combination allows for the creation of objects that change shape or properties in response to these stimuli. PCL is known for its flexibility and durability, making it suitable for a variety of applications in 4D printing. It can be used to create structures that are capable of deforming and returning to their original shape repeatedly (Rahmatabadi et al. 2023; Suriano et al. 2019; Song et al. 2022).

PCL is biocompatible and biodegradable, making it suitable for medical applications. It can be used in the manufacture of implantable devices, such as vascular stents or scaffolds for tissue engineering, where the ability to change shape over time can be beneficial. Additionally, it can be employed as structural support for other active materials in 4D printing.

6.2.2.3   Polyurethane (PU)

PU is known for its flexibility and elasticity, making it suitable for printing structures that need to change shape and adapt to different conditions. PU is a type of block polymer containing a carbamate group (-NHCOO⁻) in the molecular chain, which is composed of alternating soft and hard segments, giving it properties ranging from softness to rigidity (Zhao et al., 2023). This allows for the printing of a wide range of structures with different physical and mechanical characteristics. Due to its biocompatibility and ability to adapt to environmental changes, polyurethane can be used in printing medical devices and implants that need to adjust to internal conditions of the human body. Polyurethane is known for its resistance to wear and deterioration, making structures printed with this material more durable and suitable for prolonged use.

6.2.2.4   Liquid Crystal Elastomers (LCE)

LCE, or liquid crystal elastomers, are a unique type of smart polymer as they combine the properties of elastomers and liquid crystals. This combination allows them a variety of dynamic responses to external stimuli and exhibits properties of anisotropy and phase change when subjected to stimuli such as heat, light, or electric fields. This means they can change shape or properties in response to these stimuli, making them ideal for 4D printing. LCEs have been used to develop a variety of 4D-printed constructs, including actuators, sensors, and medical devices (Ula et al. 2018; Zeng et al. 2017).

6.2.2.5   Poly(N-Isopropylacrylamide) (pNIPAM)

The pNIPAM is a thermosensitive polymer widely used in 4D printing. This polymer exhibits a temperature-sensitive phase transition, becoming hydrophilic at lower temperatures and hydrophobic at higher temperatures (Ozturk et al. 2009). This property enables it to respond to changes in ambient temperature, altering its physical properties, which is essential in manufacturing structures that change shape over time in response to thermal stimuli.

6.2.2.6   Polyvinyl Alcohol (PVA)

Polyvinyl alcohol (PVA) acts as a support material in 4D-printing processes. It is commonly used to create temporary structures or molds that provide support during the printing of complex shapes or designs. These temporary structures are typically printed alongside the primary material using dual-extrusion or multi-material 3D printers. PVA is water-soluble and biodegradable, making it suitable for creating temporary support structures or sacrificial molds in 4D printing processes. These support structures can be easily dissolved in water after printing, leaving behind the desired 4D-printed object. PVA's versatility and compatibility with various printing techniques make it a valuable material for creating complex and intricate structures that respond dynamically to environmental stimuli (Mallakpour, Tabesh, and Hussain 2022).

6.2.2.7   Poly (Ethylene Glycol) (PEG)

PEG is known for its biocompatibility, biodegradability, and water retention capabilities, making it suitable for biomedical applications. In 4D printing, PEG can be incorporated into stimuli-responsive materials, such as hydrogels, to create structures that respond to environmental changes.

By altering the composition or manufacturing process of PEG hydrogels, it's possible to control their swelling and shrinking properties in response to specific stimuli. This enables the fabrication of structures that can change shape, size, or rigidity in real-time in response to varying environmental conditions.

By employing amide-, ester-, and thioester-linked PEG macromers functionalized with norbornene, the alteration of scaffold porosity can be readily adjusted through the combination of different ratios of these components (Miksch et al. 2022). These adaptive capabilities make PEG a popular choice for applications requiring dynamic and customized materials, such as biomedical implants, controlled drug delivery devices, and microfluidics for laboratory analysis (Luo et al. 2023; Piedade 2019; Zu et al. 2022).

6.2.2.8   Poly (Ethylene Glycol) Diacrylate (PEGDA)

PEGDA is a type of polymer commonly used in 4D printing and is a hydrogel-based material that exhibits tunable properties, such as swelling behavior and mechanical strength, making it suitable for dynamic shape-changing applications.

In 4D printing, PEGDA can be formulated into printable inks or resins. These inks or resins are typically photopolymerizable, meaning they solidify when exposed to certain types of light, such as ultraviolet (UV) light. This allows for precise control over the printing process, enabling the creation of complex 3D structures with dynamic properties.

The 4D aspect comes into play when the printed objects undergo changes in shape, size, or properties over time in response to external stimuli, such as temperature, pH level, or moisture. PEGDA-based materials can be engineered to respond to specific stimuli, enabling the design of smart structures and devices for various applications, including biomedical devices, soft robotics, and responsive textiles.

6.2.2.9 Poly (2-Hydroxyethyl Methacrylate) (PHEAA) and Poly (Methyl Methacrylate-co-Vinyl Ketone) (PMVK)

PHEAA is a polymer with potential applications in 4D printing. This polymer is known for its stimuli-responsive behavior, particularly in response to changes in environmental conditions such as temperature, pH level, or solvent composition. The polymer PHEAA-co-PMVK is an interesting material for 4D printing applications. This polymer is a copolymerization of poly(2-hydroxyethyl methacrylate) (PHEAA) and poly(methyl methacrylate-co-vinyl ketone) (PMVK), which gives unique properties to the material (NADGORNY et al. 2018).

PHEAA-co-PMVK is sensitive to changes in pH, meaning it can change shape, stiffness, or other properties in response to variations in the pH of the environment. This makes it suitable for applications where a response to specific environmental stimuli is desired.

In 4D printing, PHEAA-co-PMVK can be used to create structures that dynamically adapt to different pH conditions over time. This allows for the fabrication of objects that can change their shape or behavior in response to changes in the surrounding environment, offering a wide range of potential applications in areas such as biomaterials, biomedical devices, and soft robotics.

6.2.2.10 Alginate

Alginate is a polysaccharide derived from seaweed, often used in 3D and 4D printing due to its intriguing properties. In 4D printing, alginate can be mixed with other materials to create structures that respond to external stimuli such as changes in temperature or pH. These structures can change shape, size, or mechanical properties over time, offering potential for a variety of applications including biomedical, tissue engineering, and microfluidic devices. Alginate is particularly attractive due to its biocompatibility, biodegradability, and ability to form gels in the presence of calcium ions, facilitating the fabrication of complex and functional structures (Lee and Mooney 2012; Lai et al. 2021).

6.2.2.11 Gelatin and Collagen

Gelatin and collagen are two biomaterials commonly used in 4D printing due to their unique properties and biocompatibility. Gelatin, derived from collagen, is a hydrogel that can undergo reversible gel-sol transitions in response to changes in temperature, pH level, or ionic strength (Grogan et al. 2013). This property makes gelatin suitable for creating stimuli-responsive structures that can change shape or mechanical properties over time.

Collagen, on the other hand, is a major structural protein found in connective tissues such as skin, bones, and cartilage. It possesses excellent biocompatibility and can be used to fabricate scaffolds for tissue engineering applications. In 4D printing, collagen-based structures can be designed to degrade or remodel over time, mimicking the behavior of natural tissues.

By combining gelatin and collagen with additive manufacturing techniques, such as extrusion-based 3D printing, it is possible to create complex, bioactive structures that respond to environmental cues and have potential applications in regenerative medicine, drug delivery, and soft robotics.

6.3 SHAPE BEHAVIORS

In 4D printing, shape-changing and shape-memory behaviors refer to the ability of printed structures to alter their configuration or properties over time in response to external stimuli or to revert to a predetermined shape after being deformed, as seen in Figure 6.2.

Shape-changing behaviors can include bending, folding, twisting, expansion, contraction, and surface morphing, while shape memory refers to the ability of a material to return to its original shape after being deformed under certain conditions (Momeni et al. 2017; J. Zhou and Sheiko 2016; Patil and Sarje 2021). These features include wrinkles, creases, and buckles.

Shape-changing: Refers to the ability of a material to alter its configuration or properties in response to an external stimulus. This typically results from thermal expansion, swelling, and phase transitions, which are intrinsic properties of the material. The type of shape transformation is determined by the original material structure and is typically limited to simple affine deformations. These changes may be temporary, occurring only while the stimulus is present, and the material generally returns to its original shape after the stimulus is removed (Figure 6.2).

Shape memory: On the other hand, shape memory is the ability of a material to "remember" and return to a specific shape, even after being deformed. Shape memory transformations are not inherently encoded within a material structure and require a programming step. In this process, a sample is initially deformed by an external stimulus and then temporarily fixed into a specific shape through a vitrification

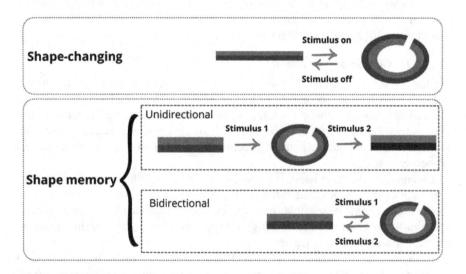

FIGURE 6.2 Shape behaviors.

process, involving crystallization, glass transition, or gelation. Essentially, the shape memory effect occurs in a two-step cycle. The first step is the programming process, where a structure is deformed from its primary shape and then held in a metastable temporary shape. The second step is the recovery process, in which the original shape can be restored through an appropriate stimulus. Additionally, it can be subdivided into two subsets: unidirectional shape memory materials and bidirectional shape memory materials (Figure 6.2).

6.4 APPLICATIONS AND ADVANTAGES

4D printing can be seen as a revolution in industries ranging from medicine to engineering. Biomimetic devices produced by 4D printing enable the simulation of biological processes and generate objects capable of environmental adaptation, offering a wide range of applications in the health sector.

Many of the structures developed by this technology can be used for grafts, biomedical devices such as smart stents, the production of artificial tissues and organs, etc. (Table 6.1). 4D bioprinting demonstrated the latest technique for producing stimuli-responsive stents of comparable size. Various 4D bioprinting techniques and materials for stents have been developed. After implantation, stents self-deform to the appropriate size and shape (Y. Zhou et al. 2021; Maity et al. 2021). Consequently, surgical interventions can be reduced.

Tissue engineering and, more specifically, skin bioprinting provide a viable therapy for severe burns, surgical wounds, and skin fragility diseases. Furthermore, it can be applied as a new drug delivery system by enabling localized drug release within the body, adjusting the transition temperature point of thermoresponsive materials closer to the physiological temperature and achieving a wide transition temperature range (Khan et al. 2022; He, Guan, and Lee 2006; Song, da Costa, and Choi 2017).

During the COVID-19 pandemic, 4D printing was essential for the development of various materials, from biomedical devices to materials that helped to prevent the spread of the disease. Among them are smart devices (face masks, hygiene products, glasses, ventilator parts, face shields, personal protective equipment), smart fabrics, microneedles, useful medical parts for infected patients and patients with diabetes, and flexible equipment for the treatment of COVID-19.

4D printing overcomes many challenges not achieved by 3D printing, with 4D printing it is possible to develop a construct capable of shaping itself according to needs under a predetermined stimulus. Currently, 4D printed devices have been used in biomedical fields, including tissue engineering, medical devices, drug delivery, as we saw previously. When using 4D printing technology, it is possible to print structures for different purposes and with complex and highly personalized geometric shapes, which can be manufactured on demand (XZhou et al. 2023). Furthermore, the possibility of printing two or more different types of materials at the same time results in implants with complex microstructures, which promotes the rapid development of precision medicine and patient recovery.

REFERENCES

Adams, A., A. Malkoc, and J. T. La Belle. 2018. "The Development of a Glucose Dehydrogenase 3D-Printed Glucose Sensor: A Proof-of-Concept Study." *Journal of Diabetes Science and Technology* 12 (1): 176–82.

Alshebly, Y. S., K. B. Mustapha, A. Zolfagharian, M. Bodaghi, M. S. Mohamed Ali, H. A. Almurib, and M. Nafea. 2022. "Bioinspired Pattern-Driven Single-Material 4D Printing for Self-Morphing Actuators." *Sustainability* 14 (16): 10141.

Barletta, M., A. Gisario, and M. Mehrpouya. 2021. "4D Printing of Shape Memory Polylactic Acid (PLA) Components: Investigating the Role of the Operational Parameters in Fused Deposition Modelling (FDM)." *Journal of Manufacturing Processes* 61: 473–80.

Bodkhe, S., and P. Ermanni. 2020. "3D Printing of Multifunctional Materials for Sensing and Actuation: Merging Piezoelectricity with Shape Memory." *European Polymer Journal* 132: 109738.

Borse, K., and P. Shende. 2023. "3D-to-4D Structures: An Exploration in Biomedical Applications." *AAPS PharmSciTech* 24 (6): 1–13.

Choi, I., S. Jang, S. Jung, S. Woo, J. Kim, C. Bak, Y. Lee, and S. Park. 2023. "A Dual Stimuli-Responsive Smart Soft Carrier Using Multi-Material 4D Printing." *Materials Horizons* 10 (9): 3668–79.

Chuayprakong, S., A. Wanamonkol, and M. Khayandee. 2020. "Programmable 4D-Printed Responsive Structures." *Key Engineering Materials* 856: 317–22. Accessed February 14, 2024. https://doi.org/10.4028/WWW.SCIENTIFIC.NET/KEM.856.317.

Cremonini, A., J. A. H. P. Sol, A. P. H. J. Schenning, S. Masiero, and M. G. Debije. 2023. "The Interplay between Different Stimuli in a 4D Printed Photo-, Thermal-, and Water-Responsive Liquid Crystal Elastomer Actuator." *Chemistry – A European Journal* 29 (36): e202300648.

Dai, S., P. Ravi, and K. C. Tam. 2008. "PH-Responsive Polymers: Synthesis, Properties and Applications." *Soft Matter* 4 (3): 435–49.

Grogan, S. P., P. H. Chung, P. Soman, P. Chen, M. K. Lotz, S. Chen, and D. D. D'Lima. 2013. "Digital Micromirror Device Projection Printing System for Meniscus Tissue Engineering." *Acta Biomaterialia* 9 (7): 7218–26.

Han, D., R. S. Morde, S. Mariani, A. A. La Mattina, E. Vignali, C. Yang, G. Barillaro, and H. Lee. 2020. "4D Printing of a Bioinspired Microneedle Array with Backward-Facing Barbs for Enhanced Tissue Adhesion." *Advanced Functional Materials* 30 (11): 1909197.

He, H., J. Guan, and J. L. Lee. 2006. "An Oral Delivery Device Based on Self-Folding Hydrogels." *Journal of Controlled Release* 110 (2): 339–46.

Hoogenboom, R. 2014. "Temperature-Responsive Polymers: Properties, Synthesis and Applications." *Smart Polymers and Their Applications*, 15–44.

Hu, Q., P. S. Katti, and Z. Gu. 2014. "Enzyme-Responsive Nanomaterials for Controlled Drug Delivery." *Nanoscale* 6 (21): 12286.

Hua, M., D. Wu, S. Wu, Y. Ma, Y. Alsaid, and X. He. 2021. "4D Printable Tough and Thermoresponsive Hydrogels." *ACS Applied Materials and Interfaces* 13 (11): 12689–97.

Huang, L., R. Jiang, J. Wu, J. Song, H. Bai, B. Li, Q. Zhao, and T. Xie. 2017. "Ultrafast Digital Printing toward 4D Shape Changing Materials." *Advanced Materials* 29 (7): 1605390.

Isaacson, A., S. Swioklo, and C. J. Connon. 2018. "3D Bioprinting of a Corneal Stroma Equivalent." *Experimental Eye Research* 173: 188–93.

Jamal, M., S. S. Kadam, R. Xiao, F. Jivan, T. M. Onn, R. Fernandes, T. D. Nguyen, and D. H. Gracias. 2013. "Bio-Origami Hydrogel Scaffolds Composed of Photocrosslinked PEG Bilayers." *Advanced Healthcare Materials* 2 (8): 1142–50.

Kang, Y., J. J. Walish, T. Gorishnyy, and E. L. Thomas. 2007. "Broad-Wavelength-Range Chemically Tunable Block-Copolymer Photonic Gels." *Nature Materials* 6 (12): 957–60.

Khan, M. S., S. A. Khan, S. Shabbir, M. Umar, S. Mohapatra, T. Khuroo, P. P. Naseef, M. S. Kuruniyan, Z. Iqbal, and M. A. Mirza. 2022. "Raw Materials, Technology, Healthcare Applications, Patent Repository and Clinical Trials on 4D Printing Technology: An Updated Review." *Pharmaceutics 2023* 15 (1): 116. Accessed February 17, 2024. https://doi.org/10.3390/PHARMACEUTICS15010116.

Lai, J., X. Ye, J. Liu, C. Wang, J. Li, X. Wang, M. Ma, and M. Wang. 2021. "4D Printing of Highly Printable and Shape Morphing Hydrogels Composed of Alginate and Methylcellulose." *Materials & Design* 205: 109699.

Lee, K. Y., and D. J. Mooney. 2012. "Alginate: Properties and Biomedical Applications." *Progress in Polymer Science* 37 (1): 106–26.

Lee, V., G. Singh, J. P. Trasatti, C. Bjornsson, X. Xu, T. N. Tran, S. S. Yoo, G. Dai, and P. Karande. 2014. "Design and Fabrication of Human Skin by Three-Dimensional Bioprinting." *Tissue Engineering. Part C, Methods* 20 (6): 473–84.

Leist, S. K., D. Gao, R. Chiou, and J. Zhou. 2017. "Investigating the Shape Memory Properties of 4D Printed Polylactic Acid (PLA) and the Concept of 4D Printing onto Nylon Fabrics for the Creation of Smart Textiles." *Virtual and Physical Prototyping* 12 (4): 290–300.

Liu, Y., F. Zhang, J. Leng, and T. W. Chou. 2021. "Microstructural Design of 4D Printed Angle-Ply Laminated Strips with Tunable Shape Memory Properties." *Materials Letters* 285: 129197.

Luo, K., L. Wang, M. X. Wang, R. Du, L. Tang, K. K. Yang, and Y. Z. Wang. 2023. "4D Printing of Biocompatible Scaffolds via In Situ Photo-Crosslinking from Shape Memory Copolyesters." *ACS Applied Materials and Interfaces* 15 (37): 44373–83. Accessed February 15, 2024. https://pubs.acs.org/doi/abs/10.1021/acsami.3c10747.

Maity, N., N. Mansour, P. Chakraborty, D. Bychenko, E. Gazit, D. Cohn, N. Maity, et al. 2021. "A Personalized Multifunctional 3D Printed Shape Memory-Displaying, Drug Releasing Tracheal Stent." *Advanced Functional Materials* 31 (50): 2108436.

Mallakpour, S., F. Tabesh, and C. M. Hussain. 2022. "A New Trend of Using Poly(Vinyl Alcohol) in 3D and 4D Printing Technologies: Process and Applications." *Advances in Colloid and Interface Science* 301: 102605.

Mao, Y., K. Yu, M. S. Isakov, J. Wu, M. L. Dunn, and H. Jerry Qi. 2015. "Sequential Self-Folding Structures by 3D Printed Digital Shape Memory Polymers." *Scientific Reports* 5 (1): 1–12.

Megdich, A., M. Habibi, and L. Laperrière. 2023. "A Review on 4D Printing: Material Structures, Stimuli and Additive Manufacturing Techniques." *Materials Letters* 337: 133977.

Mehrpouya, M., H. Vahabi, S. Janbaz, A. Darafsheh, T. R. Mazur, and S. Ramakrishna. 2021. "4D Printing of Shape Memory Polylactic Acid (PLA)." *Polymer* 230: 124080.

Melocchi, A., M. Uboldi, N. Inverardi, F. Briatico-Vangosa, F. Baldi, S. Pandini, G. Scalet, et al. 2019. "Expandable Drug Delivery System for Gastric Retention Based on Shape Memory Polymers: Development via 4D Printing and Extrusion." *International Journal of Pharmaceutics* 571: 118700.

Miksch, C. E., N. P. Skillin, B. E. Kirkpatrick, G. K. Hach, V. V Rao, T. J. White, K. S. Anseth, et al. 2022. "4D Printing of Extrudable and Degradable Poly(Ethylene Glycol) Microgel Scaffolds for Multidimensional Cell Culture." *Small* 18 (36): 2200951.

Mitkus, R., F. Cerbe, and M. Sinapius. 2022. "4D Printing Electro-Induced Shape Memory Polymers." In *Smart Materials in Additive Manufacturing, Volume 2: 4D Printing Mechanics, Modeling, and Advanced Engineering Applications*, edited by M Bodaghi and A Zolfagharian, 2nd ed., 2:19–51. Elsevier.

Momeni, F., S. M. Mehdi Hassani.N, X. Liu, and J. Ni. 2017. "A Review of 4D Printing." *Materials & Design* 122 (May): 42–79.

Mukhopadhyay, P., K. Sarkar, S. Bhattacharya, A. Bhattacharyya, R. Mishra, and P. P. Kundu. 2014. "PH Sensitive N-Succinyl Chitosan Grafted Polyacrylamide Hydrogel for Oral Insulin Delivery." *Carbohydrate Polymers* 112: 627–37. Accessed February 14, 2024. https://doi.org/10.1016/J.CARBPOL.2014.06.045.

Muzaffar, A., M. B. Ahamed, K. Deshmukh, T. Kovářík, T. Křenek, and S. K. K. Pasha. 2020. "3D and 4D Printing of PH-Responsive and Functional Polymers and Their Composites." In *3D and 4D Printing of Polymer Nanocomposite Materials: Processes, Applications, and Challenges*, 85–117. Elsevier.

Nadgorny, M., J. Collins, Z. Xiao, P. J. Scales, and L. A. Connal. 2018. "3D-Printing of Dynamic Self-Healing Cryogels with Tuneable Properties." *Polymer Chemistry* 9 (13): 1684–92.

Ozturk, N., A. Girotti, G. T. Kose, J. C. Rodríguez-Cabello, and V. Hasirci. 2009. "Dynamic Cell Culturing and Its Application to Micropatterned, Elastin-like Protein-Modified Poly(N-Isopropylacrylamide) Scaffolds." *Biomaterials* 30 (29): 5417–26.

Pandey, H., S. S. Mohol, and R. Kandi. 2022. "4D Printing of Tracheal Scaffold Using Shape-Memory Polymer Composite." *Materials Letters* 329: 133238. Accessed February 14, 2024. https://doi.org/10.1016/J.MATLET.2022.133238.

Patil, A. N., and S. H. Sarje. 2021. "Additive Manufacturing with Shape Changing/Memory Materials: A Review on 4D Printing Technology." *Materials Today: Proceedings* 44: 1744–49.

Piedade, A. P. 2019. "4D Printing: The Shape-Morphing in Additive Manufacturing." *Journal of Functional Biomaterials* 10 (1): 9.

Qiu, W., X. He, Z. Fang, Y. Wang, K. Dong, G. Zhang, X. Xu, Q. Ge, and Y. Xiong. 2023. "Shape-Tunable 4D Printing of LCEs via Cooling Rate Modulation: Stimulus-Free Locking of Actuated State at Room Temperature." *ACS Applied Materials and Interfaces* 15 (40): 47509–19.

Rahmatabadi, D., M. Aberoumand, K. Soltanmohammadi, E. Soleyman, I. Ghasemi, M. Baniassadi, K. Abrinia, M. Bodaghi, and M. Baghani. 2023. "4D Printing-Encapsulated Polycaprolactone–Thermoplastic Polyurethane with High Shape Memory Performances." *Advanced Engineering Materials* 25 (6): 2201309.

Simińska-Stanny, J., M. Nizioł, P. Szymczyk-Ziółkowska, M. Brożyna, A. Junka, A. Shavandi, and D. Podstawczyk. 2022. "4D Printing of Patterned Multimaterial Magnetic Hydrogel Actuators." *Additive Manufacturing* 49: 102506.

Song, E., T. H. da Costa, and J. W. Choi. 2017. "A Chemiresistive Glucose Sensor Fabricated by Inkjet Printing." *Microsystem Technologies* 23 (8): 3505–11.

Song, M., X. Liu, H. Yue, S. Li, and J. Guo. 2022. "4D Printing of PLA/PCL-Based Bio-Polyurethane via Moderate Cross-Linking to Adjust the Microphase Separation." *Polymer* 256: 125190.

Suriano, R., R. Bernasconi, L. Magagnin, and M. Levi. 2019. "4D Printing of Smart Stimuli-Responsive Polymers." *Journal of The Electrochemical Society* 166 (9): B3274–81. Accessed February 14, 2024. https://doi.org/10.1149/2.0411909JES/XML.

Tibbits, S. 2014. "4D Printing: Multi-Material Shape Change." *Architectural Design* 84 (1): 116–21.

Tran, T. S., R. Balu, S. Mettu, N. Roy Choudhury, and N. K. Dutta. 2022. "4D Printing of Hydrogels: Innovation in Material Design and Emerging Smart Systems for Drug Delivery." *Pharmaceuticals* 15 (10): 1282.

Ula, S. W., N. A. Traugutt, R. H. Volpe, R. R. Patel, K. Yu, and C. M. Yakacki. 2018. "Liquid Crystal Elastomers: An Introduction and Review of Emerging Technologies." *Liquid Crystals Reviews* 6 (1): 78–107.

Wang, X., X. H. Qin, C. Hu, A. Terzopoulou, X. Z. Chen, T. Y. Huang, K. Maniura-Weber, S. Pané, and B. J. Nelson. 2018. "3D Printed Enzymatically Biodegradable Soft Helical Microswimmers." *Advanced Functional Materials* 28 (45): 1804107.

Wang, Y., and X. Li. 2020. "An Accurate Finite Element Approach for Programming 4D-Printed Self-Morphing Structures Produced by Fused Deposition Modeling." *Mechanics of Materials* 151: 103628. Accessed February 14, 2024. https://doi.org/10.1016/J.MECHMAT.2020.103628.

Wang, Z., Q. Zhang, S. Long, Y. Luo, P. Yu, Z. Tan, J. Bai, et al. 2018. "Three-Dimensional Printing of Polyaniline/Reduced Graphene Oxide Composite for High-Performance Planar Supercapacitor." *ACS Applied Materials and Interfaces* 10 (12): 10437–44. Accessed January 9, 2024. https://pubs.acs.org/doi/abs/10.1021/acsami.7b19635.

Wu, Z., J. Zhao, W. Wu, P. Wang, B. Wang, G. Li, and S. Zhang. 2018. "Radial Compressive Property and the Proof-of-Concept Study for Realizing Self-Expansion of 3D Printing Polylactic Acid Vascular Stents with Negative Poisson's Ratio Structure." *Materials (Basel, Switzerland)* 11 (8): 1357.

Zeng, H., O. M. Wani, P. Wasylczyk, R. Kaczmarek, and A. Priimagi. 2017. "Self-Regulating Iris Based on Light-Actuated Liquid Crystal Elastomer." *Advanced Materials* 29 (30): 1701814.

Zhao, W., C. Yue, L. Liu, Y. Liu, and J. Leng. 2023. "Research Progress of Shape Memory Polymer and 4D Printing in Biomedical Application." *Advanced Healthcare Materials* 12 (16): 2201975.

Zhao, Y.-D., J.-H. Lai, and M. Wang. 2021. "4D Printing of Self-Folding Hydrogel Tubes for Potential Tissue Engineering Applications." *Nano Life* 11 (4): 2141001.

Zhou, J., and S. S. Sheiko. 2016. "Reversible Shape-Shifting in Polymeric Materials." *Journal of Polymer Science Part B: Polymer Physics* 54 (14): 1365–80.

Zhou, X., L. Ren, Z. Song, G. Li, J. Zhang, B. Li, Q. Wu, W. Li, L. Ren, and Q. Liu. 2023. "Advances in 3D/4D Printing of Mechanical Metamaterials: From Manufacturing to Applications." *Composites Part B: Engineering* 254: 110585.

Zhou, Y., D. Zhou, P. Cao, X. Zhang, Q. Wang, T. Wang, Z. Li, et al. 2021. "4D Printing of Shape Memory Vascular Stent Based on BCD-g-Polycaprolactone." *Macromolecular Rapid Communications* 42 (14): 2100176.

Zu, S., Z. Wang, S. Zhang, Y. Guo, C. Chen, Q. Zhang, T. Liu, Q. Liu, and Z. Zhang. 2022. "A Bioinspired 4D Printed Hydrogel Capsule for Smart Controlled Drug Release." *Materials Today Chemistry* 24: 100789.

7 Application Fields and Regulatory Aspects

7.1 INTRODUCTION

Additive manufacturing (AM) is a transformative approach developed from research and utilized in industrial production, which enables the creation of lighter, more precise, and stronger pharmaceutical products. It is yet, another technological advancement made possible by the transition from analog to digital processes. In recent decades, AM has gone beyond being a prototyping tool and evolved into a modern manufacturing solution (Awad et al. 2018; Basak 2024; Wang and Guo 2023; Chen, Xu, Kwok, et al. 2020)

3D printing can create products from 3D model data by depositing, binding, or polymerization of materials layer-by-layer until the product is obtained, as opposed to subtractive manufacturing methodologies. It has the potential to revolutionize both pharmaceutical and biomedical manufacturing by enabling highly customized products, complex geometries, and a design-driven manufacturing process (Goole and Amighi 2016; Awad et al. 2018; Elkasabgy, Mahmoud, and Maged 2020; Basit and Trenfield 2022; Tracy et al. 2023; Chakka and Chede 2023; Basak 2024).

Moreover, 4D printing is a further evolution of 3D printing. The fourth dimension here is time, implying that the 3D-printed object changes its form over time in response to environmental factors such as temperature, light, or other stimuli. These technologies open up new application areas in sectors such as medical devices and pharmaceutical dosage forms (Awad et al. 2018; Food and Drug Administration et al. 2023; Tracy et al. 2023; Wang and Guo 2023).

The printed products can be useful for the development of bioadhesive drug delivery systems and synthetic surfaces to evaluate the bioadhesiveness of systems, and also for diagnostics and theranostics (Goole and Amighi 2016; Tran et al. 2022; Food and Drug Administration et al. 2023; Wang and Guo 2023).

The advent of 3D and 4D printing technologies (3D/4D printing), together with artificial intelligence, has revolutionized numerous fields, with applications in the pharmaceutical and biomedical fields. Some key innovations are the possibility to manufcature complex products, increased personalization, and on-demand manufacturing (Food and Drug Administration et al. 2023; Grof and Štěpánek 2021; Basit and Trenfield 2022; Ramezani and Mohd Ripin 2023; Basak 2024).

The first printed solid drug delivery system (an orodispersible "tablet" containing Levetiracetam; Spritam®) was approved by the US Food and Drug Administration (FDA) in August 2015, and over the last decade there has been an increase in the number of publications on additive manufacturing of drug delivery and testing

DOI: 10.1201/9781003442363-7

systems (Lim et al. 2018; Chen, Xu, Chi Lip Kwok, et al. 2020; Mirza and Iqbal 2019).

This shows that AM can provide key advantages over traditional technologies for the preparation and production of drug delivery and testing systems (Goole and Amighi 2016; Lim et al. 2018; Basit and Trenfield 2022). Thus, this type of manufacturing is a disruptive tool for many technological areas, such as the pharmaceutical and biomedical fields. The fabrication of complex and micronized tissue scaffolds and models for drug testing systems that closely resemble in vivo conditions are possible. Actually, these technologies have opened up new possibilities for the development of personalized medicine, particularly in the creation of bioadhesive pharmaceutical systems.

Bioadhesive pharmaceutical systems refer to dosage forms that can adhere to biological surfaces, allowing for an extended time at the site of administration and also in the duration of the action. This adhesion can be achieved through various mechanisms, such as mechanical interlocking or the formation of chemical bonds. The use of AM (3D/4D printing technology) in the creation of these systems allows for a high degree of customization, enabling the creation of dosage forms tailored to the specific needs of individual patients (Goole and Amighi 2016; Elkasabgy, Mahmoud, and Maged 2020; Tran et al. 2022; Basak 2024; Chakka and Chede 2023; Wang and Guo 2023).

As discussed in previous chapters, the application of AM in the bioadhesive pharmaceuticals and biomedical fields are vast. They range from the creation of personalized dosage forms, such as tablets and capsules, to the fabrication of more complex structures, such as tissue scaffolds for regenerative medicine (Awad et al. 2018; Basak 2024; Wang and Guo 2023). The ability to precisely control the shape, size, and composition of the printed objects allows for the optimization of drug release profiles, improving the efficacy and safety of the treatment (Basit and Trenfield 2022).

The potential benefits of 3D/4D printing make it a subject of great interest for researchers, manufacturers, and policymakers in the pharmaceutical and biomedical fields (Tran et al. 2022; Wang and Guo 2023).

The high diffusion of new equipment, processes, and materials has caused excitement and accelerated the development of additive manufacturing. This scenario contributes to improving the manufacturing of personalized drug delivery platforms displaying special properties such as environmental responsiveness and bioadhesion. (Goole and Amighi 2016; Lim et al. 2018; Elkasabgy, Mahmoud, and Maged 2020; Tran et al. 2022; Wang and Guo 2023).

While these technologies hold immense promise, they also present a set of challenges that need to be addressed. These include technical issues related to material properties and printing technologies, regulatory issues, intellectual property concerns, and market concerns.

7.2   APPLICATION FIELDS AND SAFETY

AM allows for the creation of personalized bioadhesive pharmaceutical systems, tailored to the specific needs of individual patients. This can lead to improved treatment outcomes and reduced side effects (Basit and Trenfield 2022; Food and Drug Administration et al. 2023).

Bioadhesive systems display adhesion to biological surfaces, such as mucosa and skin, allowing for a prolonged period of retention at the site of administration and prolonged drug action as well. This bioadhesion can be explained by various theories, such as hydration, mechanical interlocking, or the formation of chemical interactions (Bruschi et al. 2007; Carvalho et al. 2010).

3D/4D printing technologies have found significant applications in the field of bioadhesive pharmaceutical systems such as in personalized medicine, drug delivery systems, tissue engineering, and wound healing (Goole and Amighi 2016; Elkasabgy, Mahmoud, and Maged 2020; Tran et al. 2022).

AM can be used to create bioadhesive scaffolds for tissue engineering. Bioprinting constitutes an emerging technology for AM and has numerous clinical applications in the biomedical field, enabling the production of 3D printed cell-laden constructs in a precise and controlled manner (Noroozi et al. 2023; Wang and Guo 2023). These scaffolds can mimic the natural extracellular matrix, promoting cell adhesion and tissue regeneration (Basak 2024). Moreover, printed bioadhesive platforms can be designed to adhere to specific biological surfaces, allowing for targeted drug delivery. This can improve the efficacy of the treatment and reduce systemic side effects (Goole and Amighi 2016).

AM can enable the development of bioadhesive formulations with a high degree of customization. By controlling the shape, size, and composition of the printed products, it is possible to tailor the drug release profiles to the specific needs of individual patients (Goole and Amighi 2016; Elkasabgy, Mahmoud, and Maged 2020; Basit and Trenfield 2022).

This personalization can also lead to improved treatment outcomes and reduced side effects (Elkasabgy, Mahmoud, and Maged 2020). For example, a patient displaying a chronic disease may require a slow and steady release of drugs over an extended period. Using AM, a bioadhesive platform can be developed for adhesion to the patient's body and for drug delivery at the desired site and rate. On the other hand, for acute conditions, a system can be designed to provide a rapid release of medication for immediate relief (Khaled et al. 2015; Goole and Amighi 2016).

Moreover, 4D printing technology added the dimension of time to the printing process, allowing the creation of objects that can change their shape or properties over time in response to environmental stimuli. This strategy can be useful in the design of bioadhesive systems that need to adapt to the changing conditions in the body (e.g., pH level, temperature, humidity, etc.) (M.L. Bruschi et al. 2017; Tran et al. 2022; De Souza Ferreira et al. 2016).

However, the use of AM in the development of personalized bioadhesive pharmaceutical systems also displays several challenges. During the development of the bioinks, some distinct characteristics must be considered in dependence of applications: printability, viscoelasticity, biocompatibility, bioresorbability, biodegradability, permeability, adhesion, and surface tension (Solis and Czekanski 2022; Noroozi et al. 2023; Basak 2024). Moreover, the safety of the printed materials, achieving the desired drug release profiles, their application, and navigating the regulatory landscape for personalized medicine should be considered (Noroozi et al. 2023).

Bioadhesive systems have emerged as a promising solution in the field of wound care and drug delivery. The advent of AM technologies has further expanded the potential of these systems, enabling the creation of advanced pharmaceutical wound dressings and films. The printed wound dressings can be designed to conform to the shape of the wound, ensuring optimal contact and promoting healing. They can also adhere to the wound site, providing a moist healing environment and delivering therapeutic agents to promote wound healing. In addition, 4D printing allows the creation of products that can change their shape or properties in response to environmental stimuli. For example, a 4D printed dressing could contract to apply pressure to a bleeding wound or expand to accommodate swelling (Rosseto et al. 2021; Wang and Guo 2023; Cássia Rosseto et al. 2024).

The use of bioadhesive materials from natural or synthetic origins in these systems ensures that they can adhere to the wound surface, providing a protective barrier and maintaining a moist wound environment. This not only promotes healing but also allows for the sustained release of therapeutic agents directly to the site. This targeted drug delivery can improve treatment outcomes and reduce systemic side effects (Goole and Amighi 2016; Elkasabgy, Mahmoud, and Maged 2020).

Natural polymers are often used due to their excellent biocompatibility. Together with environmentally responsive polymers, they can result in bioinks with excellent characteristics for pharmaceutical and biomedical applications. In this context, materials with a natural origin have been proposed using hyaluronic acid, collagen, gelatin, fibrin, agarose, chitosan, silk protein, and/or alginates (Tran et al. 2022; Sadeghianmaryan et al. 2022; Noroozi et al. 2023). The most used synthetic polymers for 3D/4D printing in pharmaceutical and biomedical applications are polyethylene glycol (PEG), polylactic acid (PLA), polylactic glycolic acid (PLGA), and polyethylene glycol diacrylate (PEGDA). The combination of these natural and synthetic polymers together with environmentally responsive materials (e.g., poloxamers, carbomers, and magneto-responsive materials) has been shown to be a smart strategy for the development of materials for 3D/4D printing (Tran et al. 2022; Noroozi et al. 2023; Cássia Rosseto et al. 2024; de Francisco et al. 2020).

There are safety aspects of 3D/4D printing of bioadhesive pharmaceutical systems that are of paramount importance such as material safety, quality control, regulatory compliance, and patient and environmental safety (Mirza and Iqbal 2019; Food and Drug Administration et al. 2023).

The status of AM enables to repair and produce human cells, tissues, and body parts. Actually, tissues and organs can be printed on-demand and/or on-site. Moreover, the pharmaceutical formulations are based on three fundamentals: safety, quality, and efficacy. Pharmaceutical dosage forms, such as semi-solids, films, patches, particles, and tablets, are developed to achieve these three fundamentals, which will make them effective for controlled drug delivery and safe for use. Thus, the compounds and materials used in AM must be biocompatible and safe (Lim et al. 2018; Wang and Guo 2023). This requires extensive testing and validation. The materials should not cause adverse reactions when in contact with body tissues or fluids.

All printable materials must show good biocompatibility. Some toxic acrylates are used as liquid resins for vat polymerization. However, the final printed products are biocompatible, due to the cross-linking results of large molecular-weight polymers (Wang and Guo 2023). It is also necessary to consider the risk of residual monomers leaching from the printed products. More studies are also necessary to investigate the effect of post-processes on product safety and drug stability.

Ensuring the quality and consistency of 3D/4D printed pharmaceuticals is a major challenge. Variations in the printing process can lead to inconsistencies in the final product, which can affect its safety and efficacy. Therefore, stringent quality control measures are necessary (Wang and Guo 2023).

For example, in the case of sterile products, the printing process must be conducted considering aseptic protocols. In the pharmaceutical field a final process of sterilization is very important and can often give additional assurance to the final printed product (Lim et al. 2018). However, it is necessary to keep in mind that aseptic manufacturing may be utilized during the fabrication process. The most common means of sterilization are high-temperature wet using steam (autoclave), ethylene oxide gas, hydrogen peroxide gas plasma, and gamma radiation.Sterilization by autoclave is very useful for metal surgical tools or implants. However, 3D printing technology often uses plastics or polymers that cannot be sterilized under high temperatures. Thus, the definition of the sterilization method is fundamental. Ethylene oxide gas, hydrogen peroxide gas, or gamma rays can penetrate the interior of the printed product and common packaging materials. Moreover, it is necessary to consider the other characteristics of an ideal low-temperature sterilization method such as high efficacy, fast activity, non-toxicity, adaptability, monitoring capability, and cost effectiveness (Lim et al. 2018; Chakka and Chede 2023).

It is important to highlight that printed pharmaceuticals must comply with the regulations set out by health authorities such as the FDA or EMA. This includes tests for safety, efficacy, and quality. Navigating the regulatory landscape for such novel technologies can be complex and requires a thorough understanding of the regulations.

The personalized nature of 3D/4D printed pharmaceuticals raises unique safety concerns. Ensuring the correct dosage and release profile for each patient is critical. Additionally, the risk of misuse or abuse, particularly in the context of printing controlled substances, needs to be addressed.

The environmental impact of the materials used and the waste generated during the printing process should also be considered. Using biodegradable materials and minimizing waste can contribute to environmental safety.

Each different 3D printing technology shows different advantages and limitations in terms of material choice. Understanding these technologies is very important for pharmaceutical applications.

7.3 REGULATORY ASPECTS AND MARKET

As great innovation is generally accompanied by great regulatory challenges and debate, the use of 3D/4D printing technologies in the pharmaceutical industry also raises several regulatory issues. Despite the advantages of AM, there are some challenges associated with 3D/4D technologies that make these technologies and their products different from traditional manufacturing of pharmaceuticals, for example.

The customization of dosage forms means that each printed object could be considered a new drug, raising questions about how these products should be tested and approved (Goole and Amighi 2016; Elkasabgy, Mahmoud, and Maged 2020; Basit and Trenfield 2022; Krishnan, Lakshman, and Bhargav 2023). The regulatory process of 3D/4D printing may be composed of three parts: the 3D printer, ink, and the finished product. Moreover, the pathway for approval and commercialization is not clear for each device and finished product (Parhi 2021).

AM using biological and non-biological materials that can result in regulatory challenges when compared to traditional manufacturing. Moreover, other factors may threaten the quality of formulations, such as the lack of quality control procedures for printed products at pharmacies and hospitals, low printing speed, and possible risk of cyber attacks on the computer controlling the printing process (Linares, Casas, and Caraballo 2019; Huanbutta et al. 2023; Rosch et al. 2023). Other issues during the manufacturing process may be considered and compliance with the qualification and validation iof the Good Manufacturing Practice (GMP) is fundamental.

The use of these technologies in a home setting could potentially lead to misuse, necessitating the development of regulations to ensure patient safety. The 3D/4D printed products for pharmaceutical and biomedical uses should be subordinate to regulatory requirements, such as those made by other manufacturing processes. The regulators should facilitate the development of 3D/4D technologies for pharmaceutical and biomedical applications but consider the required qualities and standards to scale the printed products for commercial manufacturing.

Several regulatory and technical issues must be considered to reach widespread pharmaceutical and biomedical applications and acceptance by the population. Regulatory laws are quite different in each country; however, most of the regulators work with periodic reports and returns, certifications, and licenses. Drug products display more stringent regulatory requirements than medical devices, surgery, education, and training tools. Moreover, the development of printed products allow quicker trials (such as studies about excipient compatibility and drug release). However, when compared with traditional dosage forms and manufacturing processes and equipments, there is a lack of clinical history and post-marketing data. Pharmacies from different sectors such as hospitals and retail will see their role change in the future (Kumar Gupta et al. 2022).

The FDA has published the Technical Considerations for Medical Devices Manufactured by AM. This mentions that the file format must be compatible with different software on the market. Patient images, design manipulation software for patient matching, digital point clouds and meshes, and machine-readable files have their specifications, coordinate systems, and default parameters, and each package has a different approach to interpreting these specifications. It is also possible to use the additive manufacturing file format (AMF) described in the ISO/ASTM 52915 specification for AMF (FDA 2017).

Thus, several key questions need to be clarified when setting out the regulatory requirement for AM pharmaceutical dosage forms (Lim et al. 2018; Krishnan, Lakshman, and Bhargav 2023). In this way, important aspects must be considered for bioadhesive inks, products and processes (Krishnan, Lakshman, and Bhargav 2023):

- quality control and good manufacturing practices;
- Risks associated with 3D printed pharmaceuticals to patients;
- Approval departments that exist, how 3D/4D printing can be regulated;
- Proposed framework of 3D/4D printing medical devices by regulators.

There is difficulty in establishing liability for damage or injury caused by the product. This liability can be imposed on any or all parties that are part of the production and supply chain, considering the issue of quality assurance, negligence, and strict liability. 3D/4D printing technologies present revolutionary implications for the pharmaceutical and biomedical fields and their consumers, in terms of the responsibility involved. Therefore, the regulation must include the pharmaceutical ink, the 3D printer, and the final product.

The different AM technologies must be recognized and regulated by regulatory agencies. It may be tedious to include all various technologies, as materials used by each technology can be quite distinct from each other (Lim et al. 2018; Krishnan, Lakshman, and Bhargav 2023).

For example, it is not clear if the inks should be regulated as a drug-device product or as a pharmaceutical ingredient, considering that the inks may be composed of drug-loaded formulations. Moreover, some inks may be toxic to humans, but the final product is not, as in the case of vat polymerization AM pharmaceutical dosage forms (Lim et al. 2018; Krishnan, Lakshman, and Bhargav 2023).

Another important aspect is the necessity for regulatory approval of clinical trials. The technology readiness level of 3D/4D printing technologies has reached studies involving animal models and clinical trials. It is fundamental to investigate the issues related to material characteristics in clinical trials to investigate the printed products in real healthcare applications (typical Phase 1 to Phase 3 clinical trials for printed products). Many clinical centers are not adopting this methodology mainly as it is not cost effective and displays segmentation troubles, alongside the challenges faced in terms of regulation (Kumar Gupta et al. 2022).

Clinical trials require 20 to 100 healthy volunteers, and 300 to 3000 volunteers with the disease/condition for Phases 1, 2, and 3 respectively (FDA 2017; Lim et al. 2018; Krishnan, Lakshman, and Bhargav 2023). However, in many cases of personalized pharmaceutical dosage forms, each product has only one single subject. It will be important to determine a fundamentally new method for fulfilling this requirement. Currently, 3D/4D printing technologies have some randomized case-control studies, most of which are published in the areas of maxillofacial surgery and orthopedics, retinal vascular disease, and gastro retentive floating pulsatile delivery systems (Kumar Gupta et al. 2022; Krishnan, Lakshman, and Bhargav 2023).

The integration of AM technologies with different dimensions of the development of the pharmaceutical or biomedical product is necessary. 3D/4D printing technologies can provide bioadhesive products in small batch sizes with highly effective dose versatility. This is very important in first-in-human trials and in preclinical studies as well. The advantage of dose flexibility is that it enables an easy, efficient, and precise means of dose evaluation and result collection. Directly after the clinical trials, it is possible to print the product for administration with neither storage nor transportation. In this context, it is not necessarily accelerated stability testing which causes an eventual delay in reaching clinical trials (Kumar Gupta et al. 2022).

The path to meeting current regulatory requirements of agencies is an uphill task that can impede the introduction of AM pharmaceutical dosage forms to the market (Lim et al. 2018). However, 3D/4D technologies and the use of stimuli-responsive materials has transformed the pharmaceutical and biomedical fields with numerous new fabrication processes, products, and revolutions. This has also contributed to the exponential growth of the bioprinting market, with a value in the range of billions of dollars (Tran et al. 2022; Noroozi et al. 2023).

7.4   MARKET, PATENTS, AND CHALLENGES

The AM market has become more diverse, and has expanded from engineering companies to start-ups and specialized 3D/4D printing companies working with materials and products for pharmaceutical and biomedical applications.

These technologies are disruptive and have some issues to be considered (Kumar Gupta et al. 2022). However, over the last two decades, more than 50,000 international patent filings for 3D printing technologies have been made worldwide. Companies from the United States, Europe, and Japan are leading the global research and intellectual protection for 3D/4D printing innovation. Public research organizations, hospitals, and universities have significantly contributed to 3D/4D printing innovation, performing approximately 12% of patent applications (EPO 2023).

Despite the advantages of 3D/4D products, they generally display a higher cost than conventional ones. This can be due to patent protection of the technology and the use of sophisticated (generally non-destructive) evaluation. Moreover, the regulatory guidelines of the AM field are still emerging, and the development process normally requires a large amount of data to get approval (Gupta et al. 2022).

Securing intellectual protection for processes, inks, and/or bioinks to print new bioadhesive systems and also human tissue/mucosa has challenges. However, the composition is the main concern.

The recent advances in this technology and the increase in the resolution of printers have also contributed to aspects of innovation that must be considered in terms of patentability of processes and products.

Considering the life sciences field, the 3D/4D technology can result in products and processes. Sometimes, the product is a biological material found in nature, and so,is not considered an invention. Whole or parts of living beings are not patentable, except for transgenic microorganisms. This can be an obstacle.

Considering the fundamentals of intellectual property and innovation, the term "natural" may refer to something that is from nature produced by nature, in which human intervention or activity is not applied. Therefore, a natural biological process occurs spontaneously in nature, and can only be discovered and not invented.

In this context, the intellectual property of 3D/4D printed products and processes should be considered when the creative process of human beings is present.

Biologic materials that are identical to naturally occurring ones but produced by printing are not eligible for protection, even in the presence of human intervention, a product resembling its natural reference is not subject to patent in many countries (EPO 2023).

A report published by the European Patent Office (EPO) in September 2023 showed that 3D printing filings surged in the past decade. From 2013 to 2020, the number of international patents in 3D printing increased at a mean annual rate of 26.3%. This rate is about eight times faster than for all technology fields combined in the same period which was 3.3% (EPO 2023). Among them, are several patents related to materials, inks, and printed bioadhesive systems. Together, these patent families can conduce in the near future to printed bioadhesive formulations in the market.

As already discussed, AM enables mass customization, avoiding some traditional technical restrictions to the industrial production process and can reduce waste. The pharmaceutical and biomedical sectors have attracted most of the 3D printing applications.

From 2001 to 2020, one-fifth of all international patent filings published were in the health and medical sectors (about 10,000), largely explained by the advances in pharmaceutical and biomedical applications for 3D printing. In this scenario, the AM market displays strong growth, with industry revenue tripling from USD 6 billion in 2016 to USD 18 billion (EUR 16.17 billion) in 2022 (EPO 2023).

It is important to point out the importance that 3D printing technologies played during the COVID-19 pandemic. They enabled the switch to local production, reducing dependence on international supply chains. Projections suggest the market could exceed USD 50 billion by 2028 (EPO 2023).

7.5 CONCLUSIONS AND PERSPECTIVES

AM was developed for rapid prototyping. Nowadays, it has displayed an important improvement in its speed, precision, and accuracy, which has enabled upscaling into industrial fabrication. Thus, using AM in large-scale manufacturing is a reality. Traditional manufacturing of solid dosage forms, such as tablets, can fabricate up to 1.6 million tablets per hour. This amount far exceeds what a 3D printer can currently do. However, the pharmaceutical dosage forms created by AM can display unique characteristics, which are not possible to be obtained by high-speed tableting. Considering that the speed, quality, and material for AM are improving quickly, new opportunities will arise that take AM ever closer to mass production.

3D/4D printing technologies hold great promise for the future of the pharmaceutical industry. However, the realization of this potential will require careful consideration of the associated regulatory aspects to ensure that these technologies are used safely and effectively. Careful consideration must be given to the safety aspects to ensure the wellbeing of patients. Collaborative efforts from scientists, engineers, clinicians, and regulatory bodies are needed (Noroozi et al. 2023). Moreover, several countries have discussed and proposed a national coordination for the adoption and promotion of AM (Lim et al. 2018).

While there are challenges to be overcome, 3D/4D printing holds great promise in the creation of personalized bioadhesive pharmaceutical systems, potentially revolutionizing the field of drug delivery and paving the way for a new era of personalized medicine. As research in this area continues to advance, we can look forward to a future where personalized, adaptive bioadhesive medicines are the norm rather than the exception.

REFERENCES

Awad, Atheer, Sarah J. Trenfield, Alvaro Goyanes, Simon Gaisford, and Abdul W. Basit. 2018. "Reshaping Drug Development Using 3D Printing." *Drug Discovery Today* 23 (8): 1547–55. https://doi.org/10.1016/j.drudis.2018.05.025.

Basak, Sayan. 2024. "Is 4D Printing at the Forefront of Transformations in Tissue Engineering and Beyond?" *Biomedical Materials & Devices*, January. https://doi.org/10.1007/s44174-024-00161-9.

Basit, Abdul W., and Sarah J. Trenfield. 2022. "3D Printing of Pharmaceuticals and the Role of Pharmacy." *Pharmaceutical Journal*. https://doi.org/10.1211/PJ.2022.1.135581.

Bruschi, M. L., F. B. Borghi-Pangoni, M. V. Junqueira, S. B. de Souza Ferreira, and J. B. da Silva. 2017. "Environmentally Responsive Systems for Drug Delivery." *Recent Patents on Drug Delivery and Formulation* 11 (2). https://doi.org/10.2174/187221131166617 0328151455.

Bruschi, Marcos L., David S. Jones, Heitor Panzeri, Maria P. D. Gremião, Osvaldo de Freitas, and Elza H. G. Lara. 2007. "Semisolid Systems Containing Propolis for the Treatment of Periodontal Disease: In Vitro Release Kinetics, Syringeability, Rheological, Textural, and Mucoadhesive Properties." *Journal of Pharmaceutical Sciences* 96 (8): 2074–89.

Carvalho, Flávia Chiva, Marcos Luciano Bruschi, Raul Cesar Evangelista, and Maria Palmira Daflon Gremião. 2010. "Mucoadhesive Drug Delivery Systems." *Brazilian Journal of Pharmaceutical Sciences*. https://doi.org/10.1590/S1984-82502010000100002.

Cássia Rosseto, Hélen, Lucas de Alcântara Sica de Toledo, Rafaela Said dos Santos, Ana Julia Viana Ferreira, Lidiane Vizioli de Castro Hoshino, Bento Pereira Cabral Júnior, Gustavo Braga, et al. 2024. "Effect of Propolis and Polymer Content on Mechanical, Bioadhesive and Biological Properties of Nanostructured Film Forming Platforms for Topical Drug Delivery." *Journal of Molecular Liquids* 395 (February): 123878. https://doi.org/10.1016/j.molliq.2023.123878.

Chakka, L. R. Jaidev, and Shanthi Chede. 2023. "3D Printing of Pharmaceuticals for Disease Treatment." *Frontiers in Medical Technology* 4 (January). https://doi.org/10.3389/fmedt.2022.1040052.

Chen, Grona, Yihua Xu, Philip Chi Lip Kwok, and Lifeng Kang. 2020. "Pharmaceutical Applications of 3D Printing." *Additive Manufacturing* 34 (August): 101209. https://doi.org/10.1016/j.addma.2020.101209.

Elkasabgy, Nermeen A., Azza A. Mahmoud, and Amr Maged. 2020. "3D Printing: An Appealing Route for Customized Drug Delivery Systems." *International Journal of Pharmaceutics* 588 (October): 119732. https://doi.org/10.1016/j.ijpharm.2020.119732.

EPO, European Patent Office. 2023. "Patent Filings in 3D Printing Grew Eight Times Faster than Average of All Technologies in Last Decade." https://www.epo.org/en/news-events/news/patent-filings-3d-printing-grew-eight-times-faster-average-all-technologies-last#:~:text=in last decade-,Patent filings in 3D printing grew eight times faster than,all technologies in last decade&text=Areportpubli.

FDA. 2017. "Technical Considerations for Additive Manufactured Devices." http://www.fda.gov/downloads/MedicalDevices/DeviceRegulationandGuidance/GuidanceDocuments/UCM499809.pdf.

Food and Drug Administration, Andrea Gazzaniga, Anastasia Foppoli, Matteo Cerea, Luca Palugan, Micol Cirilli, Saliha Moutaharrik, et al. 2023. "Pharmaceutical Applications of 3D Printing Technology: Current Understanding and Future Perspectives." *International Journal of Pharmaceutics* 15 (2): 586–96. https://doi.org/10.3390/pharmaceutics15010116.

Francisco, L. M. B. de, D. Pinto, H. C. Rosseto, L. D. A. S. de Toledo, R. S. dos Santos, P. J. C. D. Costa, M. B. P. P. Oliveira, B. Sarmento, F. Rodrigues, and M. L. Bruschi. 2020. "Design and Characterization of an Organogel System Containing Ascorbic Acid Microparticles Produced with Propolis By-Product." *Pharmaceutical Development and Technology* 25 (1). https://doi.org/10.1080/10837450.2019.1669643.

Goole, Jonathan, and Karim Amighi. 2016. "3D Printing in Pharmaceutics: A New Tool for Designing Customized Drug Delivery Systems." *International Journal of Pharmaceutics* 499 (1–2): 376–94. https://doi.org/10.1016/j.ijpharm.2015.12.071.

Grof, Zdeněk, and František Štěpánek. 2021. "Artificial Intelligence Based Design of 3D-Printed Tablets for Personalised Medicine." *Computers & Chemical Engineering* 154 (November): 107492. https://doi.org/10.1016/j.compchemeng.2021.107492.

Huanbutta, Kampanart, Kanokporn Burapapadh, Pornsak Sriamornsak, and Tanikan Sangnim. 2023. "Practical Application of 3D Printing for Pharmaceuticals in Hospitals and Pharmacies." *Pharmaceutics* 15 (7): 1877. https://doi.org/10.3390/pharmaceutics15071877.

Khaled, Shaban A., Jonathan C. Burley, Morgan R. Alexander, Jing Yang, and Clive J. Roberts. 2015. "3D Printing of Five-in-One Dose Combination Polypill with Defined Immediate and Sustained Release Profiles." *Journal of Controlled Release* 217 (November): 308–14. https://doi.org/10.1016/j.jconrel.2015.09.028.

Krishnan, Anirudh Venkatraman, S. Anush Lakshman, and Aishwarya Bhargav. 2023. "3D Printing and Regulatory Considerations." In *3D & 4D Printing Methods for Pharmaceutical Manufacturing and Personalised Drug Delivery*, 45–68. https://doi.org/10.1007/978-3-031-34119-9_3.

Kumar Gupta, Dipak, Mohd Humair Ali, Asad Ali, Pooja Jain, Md. Khalid Anwer, Zeenat Iqbal, and Mohd. Aamir Mirza. 2022. "3D Printing Technology in Healthcare: Applications, Regulatory Understanding, IP Repository and Clinical Trial Status." *Journal of Drug Targeting* 30 (2): 131–50. https://doi.org/10.1080/1061186X.2021.1935973.

Lim, Seng Han, Himanshu Kathuria, Justin Jia Yao Tan, and Lifeng Kang. 2018. "3D Printed Drug Delivery and Testing Systems — a Passing Fad or the Future?" *Advanced Drug Delivery Reviews* 132 (July): 139–68. https://doi.org/10.1016/j.addr.2018.05.006.

Linares, Vicente, Marta Casas, and Isidoro Caraballo. 2019. "Printfills: 3D Printed Systems Combining Fused Deposition Modeling and Injection Volume Filling. Application to Colon-Specific Drug Delivery." *European Journal of Pharmaceutics and Biopharmaceutics* 134 (January): 138–43. https://doi.org/10.1016/j.ejpb.2018.11.021.

Mirza, Mohd. A., and Zeenat Iqbal. 2019. "3D Printing in Pharmaceuticals: Regulatory Perspective." *Current Pharmaceutical Design* 24 (42): 5081–83. https://doi.org/10.2174/1381612825666181130163027.

Noroozi, Reza, Zia Ullah Arif, Hadi Taghvaei, Muhammad Yasir Khalid, Hossein Sahbafar, Amin Hadi, Ali Sadeghianmaryan, and Xiongbiao Chen. 2023. "3D and 4D Bioprinting Technologies: A Game Changer for the Biomedical Sector?" *Annals of Biomedical Engineering* 51 (8): 1683–712. https://doi.org/10.1007/s10439-023-03243-9.

Parhi, Rabinarayan. 2021. "A Review of Three-Dimensional Printing for Pharmaceutical Applications: Quality Control, Risk Assessment and Future Perspectives." *Journal of Drug Delivery Science and Technology* 64 (August): 102571. https://doi.org/10.1016/j.jddst.2021.102571.

Ramezani, Maziar, and Zaidi Mohd Ripin. 2023. "4D Printing in Biomedical Engineering: Advancements, Challenges, and Future Directions." *Journal of Functional Biomaterials* 14 (7): 347. https://doi.org/10.3390/jfb14070347.

Rosch, Moritz, Tobias Gutowski, Michael Baehr, Jan Eggert, Karl Gottfried, Christopher Gundler, Sylvia Nürnberg, Claudia Langebrake, and Adrin Dadkhah. 2023. "Development of an Immediate Release Excipient Composition for 3D Printing via Direct Powder Extrusion in a Hospital." *International Journal of Pharmaceutics* 643 (August): 123218. https://doi.org/10.1016/j.ijpharm.2023.123218.

Rosseto, Hélen Cássia, Lucas de Alcântara Sica de Toledo, Rafaela Said dos Santos, Lizziane Maria Belloto de Francisco, Camila Félix Vecchi, Elisabetta Esposito, Rita Cortesi, and Marcos Luciano Bruschi. 2021. "Design of Propolis-Loaded Film Forming Systems for Topical Administration: The Effect of Acrylic Acid Derivative Polymers." *Journal of Molecular Liquids* 322 (January): 114514. https://doi.org/10.1016/j.molliq.2020.114514.

Sadeghianmaryan, Ali, Saman Naghieh, Zahra Yazdanpanah, Hamed Alizadeh Sardroud, N. K. Sharma, Lee D. Wilson, and Xiongbiao Chen. 2022. "Fabrication of Chitosan/Alginate/Hydroxyapatite Hybrid Scaffolds Using 3D Printing and Impregnating Techniques for Potential Cartilage Regeneration." *International Journal of Biological Macromolecules* 204 (April): 62–75. https://doi.org/10.1016/j.ijbiomac.2022.01.201.

Solis, Daphene Marques, and Aleksander Czekanski. 2022. "3D and 4D Additive Manufacturing Techniques for Vascular-like Structures – A Review." *Bioprinting* 25 (March): e00182. https://doi.org/10.1016/j.bprint.2021.e00182.

Souza Ferreira, Sabrina Barbosa De, Talita Dias Moço, Fernanda Belincanta Borghi-Pangoni, Mariana Volpato Junqueira, and Marcos Luciano Bruschi. 2016. "Rheological, Mucoadhesive and Textural Properties of Thermoresponsive Polymer Blends for Biomedical Applications." *Journal of the Mechanical Behavior of Biomedical Materials* 55 (March): 164–78. https://doi.org/10.1016/j.jmbbm.2015.10.026.

Tracy, Timothy, Lei Wu, Xin Liu, Senping Cheng, and Xiaoling Li. 2023. "3D Printing: Innovative Solutions for Patients and Pharmaceutical Industry." *International Journal of Pharmaceutics* 631 (January): 122480. https://doi.org/10.1016/j.ijpharm.2022.122480.

Tran, Tuan Sang, Rajkamal Balu, Srinivas Mettu, Namita Roy Choudhury, and Naba Kumar Dutta. 2022. "4D Printing of Hydrogels: Innovation in Material Design and Emerging Smart Systems for Drug Delivery." *Pharmaceuticals* 15 (10): 1282. https://doi.org/10.3390/ph15101282.

Wang, Huanhui, and Jianpeng Guo. 2023. "Recent Advances in 4D Printing Hydrogel for Biological Interfaces." *International Journal of Material Forming* 16 (5): 55. https://doi.org/10.1007/s12289-023-01778-9.

8 Concluding Remarks

Additive manufacturing is especially important and effective in several industrial areas, but it presents some limitations and challenges that need to be overcome. The way the product is printed can influence the quality of surface accuracy, height, and volume. Therefore, specialized labor in 3D printing is extremely necessary.

Bioadhesive products to be used in the pharmaceutical and/or biomedical field need to present specific characteristics such as quality, safety, and efficacy. Specialized and qualified people will enable the development of well-designed structures.

Another key point to highlight is the need to have knowledge about the types of printers, knowing how to use appropriate programs for each type of application, as well as the type of materials that can be printed. The different printing techniques play a fundamental role in obtaining the structure, having their own characteristics and different material needs. Therefore, choosing the appropriate printer is essential.

Prior knowledge of active and inert pharmaceutical ingredients is essential. The chemical composition, as well as the physical–chemical properties and geometric characteristics of the material, will influence the control of the temporal and spatial release of the drug from the bioadhesive system.

Individualized therapy is a particularly important advantage of printed medicines, and the use of bioadhesive material can contribute to obtaining systems according to the patient's preferences and needs.

In this sense, there are a variety of types of printers and printing techniques. In the area of bioadhesive materials, it is no different and many bioadhesives of natural or synthetic origin can be used. Common materials that are already used in food and medicine production and pharmaceutical ingredients (e.g., gelatin, collagen, alginate, gums, cellulose derivatives, and chitosan) are utilized. However, each printing technique and type of printer may limit the material or ink to be used.

Biodegradable, biocompatible, and non-toxic materials are always the pursuit of the research and development sector of products for human and animal use. The bioadhesive, mechanical, and rheological properties of these materials are especially important during the design and printing of systems. It is important to always keep in mind that additive manufacturing makes it possible to offer the patient a more individualized and personalized treatment. Thus, a bioadhesive system obtained by 3D printing makes it possible to adjust the dose according to the patient's individual needs. It is possible to change the size and format of the system to be printed depending on the drug concentration and dosage to be used.

It is also possible to develop and print true bioadhesive drug release platforms, seeking spatial and temporal control of the biologically active agent.

3D printing of a new bioadhesive system depends on the polymers used, which will enable it to adhere effectively to the skin or mucosa. The regulatory sector is another issue to be highlighted. The lack of laws and regulations is a challenge to be

  DOI: 10.1201/9781003442363-8

faced. Bioadhesive materials to be used in additive manufacturing appear to be very promising for various pharmaceutical and biomedical applications. Both inputs and printed products must meet strict quality and safety criteria. However, the lack of supervision and regulation can hinder the sector's rapid growth.

International regulatory agencies, such as the FDA and EMA, have sought to instruct and regulate the market. Regulatory aspects, which guarantee the quality of printed systems during development until the product is obtained, are fundamental. This is a beginning, where basic considerations about additive manufacturing are addressed.

Even considering the many advantages of additive manufacturing (3D and 4D printing) for obtaining bioadhesive systems, ensuring the effectiveness and safety of printed devices is fundamental. Materials and printing conditions must be optimized. The choice of input is a critical factor in ensuring quality, effectiveness, and safety.

Furthermore, 4D printing is revolutionary in enabling the printed product to respond and adapt to the environment. Many of the structures developed by this technique are already being applied in biomedicine and pharmacy, with a consequent reduction in surgical invasiveness, for example.

Bioprinting has also enabled the development of increasingly effective bioadhesive and biocompatible materials and systems. The use in tissue engineering and in obtaining implants with complex microstructures has provided the rapid development of precision medicine and patient recovery.

Thus, additive manufacturing has enabled important improvements in speed, precision, and accuracy, also enabling upscaling for the industrial manufacturing of pharmaceutical and biomedical products. With improvements in terms of production/printing speed, additive manufacturing will get closer and closer to mass production.

There are challenges to overcome, but 3D/4D printing of bioadhesive materials and systems is a reality and shows extremely promising paths. With the advancement of research in this field and the accumulation of knowledge and technological innovations, it is possible to envisage a promising future for printed bioadhesive materials and systems that are increasingly personalized to the needs of the patient and their therapy.

Index